The

YOGA
MIND

The

YOGA
MIND

52 ESSENTIAL PRINCIPLES

OF YOGA PHILOSOPHY TO
DEEPEN YOUR PRACTICE

RINA JAKUBOWICZ

ROCKRIDGE
PRESS

For my beloved guru,
Swamiji (Swami Parthasarathy).
Without your guidance, I'd have no road to
walk on nor words to write in this book.

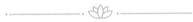

For my beloved husband, Eric Paskel,
and our colorful moments of laughter, tears,
wisdom, and choosing the higher road.
May we keep cruising upward.

CONTENTS

The Eight Limbs of Yoga

Practice

Chakras

Hatha Yoga Styles

INTRODUCTION

This book you are holding is a compilation of almost 20 years of self-study, reflection, research, questioning, and determination in a short, simplified format. It's the kind of book I would have appreciated when I started studying Yoga philosophy to help me understand the dense and overly academic translation of the ancient texts.

I became inspired to learn the inner workings of philosophical texts after reading Benjamin Hoff's *The Tao of Pooh* at 16 years old. It ignited the spark to reflect on the deeper workings of who I am and how I relate to the world. I wanted to learn more, but I didn't know where to start. I began my physical yoga practice a few years later and came to find the *Yoga Sutras of Patañjali*, which promised Enlightenment and realization of one's pure Self for everlasting freedom and happiness. I didn't know what this meant, but I knew instinctively that it was true. I immediately became a seeker of this truth and dove deep into the teachings. This was only the beginning of my search.

This book will help you become better educated to make an informed, more conscious decision about which path and direction your yoga can go. This book is by no means meant to be the end of your search but rather a map to guide your journey.

I started practicing yoga in 2000, when there wasn't a massive amount of media about yoga available. True seekers had to hunt for the truth.

Over the next 17 years, I hunted. I dedicated myself to learning and understanding an entirely new perspective and approach to life beyond this physical plane, a perspective that promises everlasting joy and happiness *and* lives within me already. It is an approach that makes my life fuller and makes me a better person, helping me deal with my angers and fears in a healthy way.

After many years of studying and applying the principles as best I could, I had a feeling this system couldn't take me to what Yoga promises: eternal bliss and Enlightenment. I saw its weaknesses and knew there were missing pieces. As a yoga teacher, I felt bad sharing these teachings with my students, knowing they couldn't reach Enlightenment.

Thus I kept searching and hunting.

Finally I found the system of Vedanta with my present and forever teacher, Swami A. Parthasarathy, who has dedicated 60 years of his life to seeking and studying the truth. He handed me the missing piece of this elaborate and perfect puzzle—the inclusion of the intellect, which we don't know we have, and the difference between it and the mind, and how it relates to my world. The intellect can also be called "the yoga mind," which is not to be confused with the mind itself. In this book I'll explain the difference between the two. In general, you'll want to strengthen your yoga mind and weaken your regular mind in order to get closer to the truth and the ultimate goal of yoga philosophy: Self-Realization. With this knowledge, we all have a chance at learning how to live our lives fully and happily.

I can now present this philosophy, with all its limbs and extensions, to you in a simple and comprehensible manner—one you can take and digest for yourself.

Whenever you open this book—to read one topic or the whole book—I hope you gain clarity on some basic concepts and how they relate to your daily life. Ideally, you'll be motivated to learn and question more. You have here in your hands all the basic aspects of Yoga philosophy and a guide to continue your search. These teachings are priceless, and it's an honor to share them with you. However, you shouldn't take what I say as truth; discover it for yourself. That is when knowledge becomes wisdom. Taste, chew, swallow, digest, and take in the nutrients for yourself.

This book is for someone who already practices yoga and is intrigued by its complex traditional origins but appreciates when they are explained in a simple, conversational way. It is written so you can select a topic you are curious about and read about it at random, or you can read the book cover to cover, building on your knowledge as you go. More important, it's for someone who is curious, who questions, and who is willing to find the answers for themselves.

Note: Some Sanskrit words and pose names are spelled phonetically and some do not use the correct Sanskrit characters. For example, "dristi" is normally spelled with a diacritic on the "s" so that it's pronounced as a "sh" sound. I changed it to "drishti" for ease of pronunciation.

ETERNAL BLISS = TURIYA = ENLIGHTENMENT = SELF-REALIZATION = SAMADHI = LIBERATION =

ABSOLUTE REALITY = THE SELF = BRAHMAN = ATMAN = GOD = PURE CONSCIOUSNESS = ABSOLUTE TRUTH = ABSOLUTE REALITY =

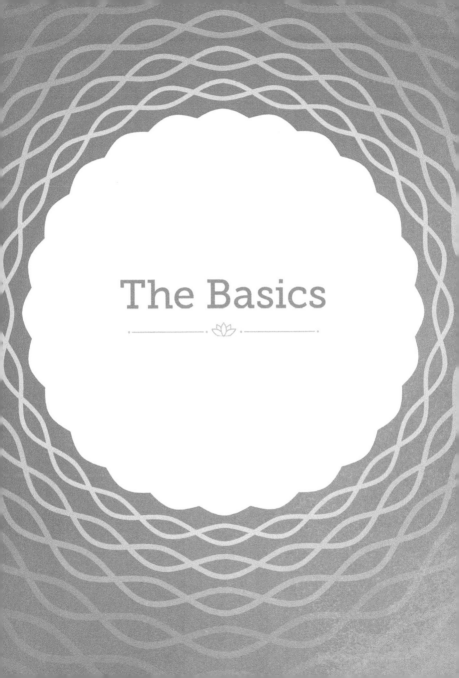

The Basics

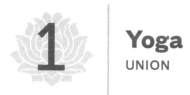

Yoga
UNION

MEANING *Yoga* is translated as "union" and is defined as the science of realizing one's true Self (see page 29), leading one to Enlightenment. *Are you scratching your head already?*

SIGNIFICANCE Discovering Yoga, a.k.a. Self-realization, is what the ancient teachings say is your number-one business in this life, giving you purpose and meaning.

EFFECT Traditionally, Yoga promises lasting happiness. It removes ignorance and thus creates the effect of eternal peace. *Sign me up!*

Yoga is the union of matter (body, mind, and intellect) with its original nature—Spirit. When you unite with the Self and no longer identify with the limitations of your body, mind, and intellect, you experience *nonduality*, known as absolute truth. This eliminates all illusions of worldly duality, known as relative truth.

If you are confused, it's okay. There is much to learn—patience is key.

This eventual union begins with unlearning what you have already learned to be "true," and is aided by the practices of self-reflection and devotion ... to a higher ideal ... to the Divine ... to Brahman ... to the Self—selfless actions, ethical principles, etc. It's the process of questioning what you've been taught from childhood and discovering for yourself whether it's true or not.

Although physical postures and breath control assist the body in becoming healthy, they alone cannot lead to Enlightenment. *Sorry. I know we all wish we could touch our toes and become enlightened, but it's not that simple.* These physical practices only help heal and purify our matter. A true yogi is a seeker of absolute truth above all else.

Still confused? Don't worry. There are many topics to explore, and we have a lifetime to do it.

Grab your journal and pen. You're going to learn to unlearn. Unlearning is the process of reflecting upon beliefs you've learned and asking, "Is this true in absolute reality?"

Absolute reality means there are no prejudices, opinions, or perceptions. For example, let's say I was taught eggplants are awful because my dad hated them. Does this mean they are awful? If I remove my prejudices, I will see that eggplants are neither awful nor delicious. It depends on the person—implying it is relative truth. If I can remove myself from my own and other's opinions, I can begin to understand the basis of absolute reality.

Write your own example of something you've learned, and go through this questioning process. *See what you can unlearn.*

Yoga isn't about standing on your head.
It's about getting your head out of your ass.

—Eric Paskel
PHILOSOPHER AND PSYCHOTHERAPIST

---

2 Namaste

BOWING TO YOU

MEANING *Namaste* is colloquially described as "the light within me honors and loves the light within you." The word *light* may be replaced with Spirit, Divinity, or Pure Consciousness.

SIGNIFICANCE Saying "Namaste" is an expression of honor and respects the other person as being made of the same Pure Consciousness as you. *Isn't that beautiful?*

EFFECT The effect of saying and hearing "Namaste" is to feel a sense of union, compassion, and acknowledgment regardless of external differences.

"Namaste" is said with one's hands in prayer position in front of the heart and with a slight bow to the head. The intention behind saying "Namaste" has changed with its modernization and mass exposure. It is now said at the end of yoga class, prompted by the teacher to the students, as a form of mutual respect and a sign that class is over. Additionally, having students say it to one another after class adds a special touch of community and connection. *This helps us realize we aren't alone and moves us beyond ourselves.*

In India, "Namaste" is a general greeting, like a casual "hello," and is not necessarily part of a yoga class. Adding "Namaste" to the end of a yoga class is something the West has applied.

"Namaste" to you, curious reader, as you embark on this journey through yoga philosophy. I honor and love you.

There is so much good in the worst of us,
and so much bad in the best of us,
that it ill behooves any of us
to find fault with the rest of us.

—James Truslow Adams
AMERICAN WRITER AND HISTORIAN

PRACTICE

Sit comfortably with your spine long and your hands in prayer position in front of your heart. Close your eyes. Visualize someone you love. Feel that warmth and light in your heart. Bow your head and say "Namaste" to the person, genuinely, three times.

Now think of a person who gets on your nerves. You might find this challenging, but visualize that person while sending the same light and warmth, repeating "Namaste" three times. See if you can feel that oneness—of being made from the same Pure Consciousness (see page 29)—instead of focusing on your differences. *This will be hard at first, and you might resist, but give it a shot. You have nothing to lose and so much to gain.*

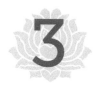

3

Vedanta
END OF KNOWLEDGE

MEANING *Vedanta* is scientific knowledge explaining how to have both an active and peaceful life. *Yes, you can have both!*

SIGNIFICANCE Learning Vedanta is like owning a user's manual to life. You'll be able to handle any challenge with grace and objectivity. *Amen!*

EFFECT Studying and practicing Vedanta on a daily basis brings about understanding, calmness, and stress reduction in all areas of your life. *Let's Vedanta!*

Vedanta is a way of living and a manual for life. It was originally founded between 1800 and 1000 BCE. Yoga masters at that time noticed that, while the external world was being perfected, people were still suffering and experiencing stress. They deduced that the objects weren't the problem, but rather the subjects themselves. The yogis decided to focus on studying themselves as subjects instead of obsessing or attaching to objects of the world.

Thus, Vedanta is the systemized study of oneself, translating to the "end of knowledge"—implying this knowledge gained is all one needs to learn for a harmonious and full life.

Truths and laws were discovered relevant to all beings regardless of race, religion, education, etc. Vedanta guides you to discovering your true essence—the Pure Self within, a.k.a. Spirit (see page 29).

Vedanta cries out to one and all:
You are making a veritable hell of the world.
Acquire this chaste knowledge. You will then
turn the world into a heaven.

—Swami A. Parthasarathy

Stand tall. Lift your left leg and place the sole of your left foot on the inside of your right thigh for Vriksha-sana, Tree Pose; if you need a modification, put the left heel onto the right ankle and keep your toes on the floor for more balance. *Note:* Do not put the sole of your foot directly on the knee—either above or below is okay. Bring your hands into prayer position in front of your heart. Hold for 5 breaths and ask yourself, "Who is doing this pose?" Go to the deepest layer of the answer. Don't just say, "I am." Who is that "I"?

After 5 breaths, switch sides. Hold the right side for 5 breaths and ask yourself, "What is creating balance in this pose?" Again, take away the externals—like the obvious answer, your muscles—and see what arises. We are only creating the ability to question here, not necessarily finding the answers. *Humor me, please. You may unlock something within yourself—possibly wonder and curiosity.*

4

Bhagavad Gita
SONG OF GOD

MEANING One of the most ancient Hindu texts, the Bhagavad Gita embodies the theme of realizing one's true essential nature in a conversation between Arjuna and Krishna.

SIGNIFICANCE The Bhagavad Gita contains the guidelines for understanding how to seek and find the truth within oneself. *You can't handle the truth! Or can you?*

EFFECT The Gita promises a peaceful and harmonious life. If you follow just one of the guidelines fully, you can get to the truth.

The Bhagavad Gita, written between 1000 and 500 BCE, translates to "Song of God" and is the philosophical part of a greater text called the *Mahabharata*, written by the sage Vyasa. The story represents the battle within ourselves—between the higher and lower qualities. It's a conversation between Arjuna, a warrior (the lower qualities), and Krishna, an incarnation of Brahman (the higher qualities; see page 29).

Arjuna, paralyzed on the battlefield, realizes he has to fight his old teacher and his family, who have terrorized the kingdom. His fight is righteous, but his attachments to his past make it hard for him to take action and do his duty. This battle is a parallel to the battle in our own lives. Our daily interactions and challenges are our battlefield, where we are constantly confronted with choosing the higher or lower options. The Bhagavad Gita helps us understand how to reach for the higher option—continually and consciously.

Let man lift himself by himself,
let him not lower himself; his self alone
is his friend, his self alone is his enemy.

—Vyasa
BHAGAVAD GITA, CHAPTER 6, VERSE 5

PRACTICE

Grab your journal and a pen. Sitting quietly, somewhere that helps you reflect, visualize a difficult decision you have to make. Make a list of pros and cons related to the decision. Using the pros and cons list, visualize yourself making one decision and imagine the effect it could have in the near and far future on everyone around you—including yourself. Consider: Does it serve others and yourself? Does it serve yourself and harm others? Does it harm everyone, including yourself?

Now do the same for the remaining choices. Going through the process of considering how your actions affect others is the first step to becoming more aware of your service and purpose in life.

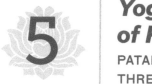

Yoga Sutras of Patañjali

PATAÑJALI'S YOGA THREADS

MEANING The *Yoga Sutras of Patañjali* is the main text from Raja Yoga—the Eight-Limbed Path that provides guidelines for daily living. Consider it the abridged version of Yoga philosophy!

SIGNIFICANCE Most beginner yogis use this system as their first guide when transitioning principles from the mat to life off the mat.

EFFECT Studying the *Yoga Sutras* can provide insight into the nature of how your mind functions. The mind is the most complex and powerful piece of equipment you have. *Better to use it wisely.*

The *Yoga Sutras* were written by Maharishi Patañjali between 500 BCE and 200 CE. They were verbally passed down to students, who wrote down their recollections of the teachings. A *sutra* is translated as a "thread" because it is meant to be strung together to create a seamless message.

The *Yoga Sutras* is divided into four portions: Contemplation, Practice, Accomplishments, and Absoluteness. The first two portions are more practical and accessible; the final two portions are abstract, making it challenging for the student to progress.

The second sutra is the most important. It gives both the definition and practice of Yoga according to Patañjali. It states, "*Yogas citta vritti nirodhah*," meaning, "Yoga is the cessation of the modifications of the mind-stuff." It explains that once you control your mind and stop it from fluctuating with desires and emotions, you will experience Yoga. *Easier said than done.*

For those who have an intense urge for Spirit
and wisdom, it sits near them, waiting.

—Patañjali
YOGA SUTRAS OF PATAÑJALI

PRACTICE

The second sutra of the *Yoga Sutras of Patañjali* says, "Yoga is the cessation of the modifications of the mind-stuff." Sutra 12 explains how to cease these thoughts, saying, "These mental modifications are restrained by practice and nonattachment." Although this is a general explanation, it does force one to reflect on how these two basic suggestions are the most challenging. Nowadays people want instant results, so practicing something for an unending amount of time can seem pointless and frustrating. Additionally, we, as a society, are driven by results, and Patañjali suggests we act without expecting anything in return—nonattachment.

In your journal, write down your observations about how this sutra might alter your daily activities.

Vedanta

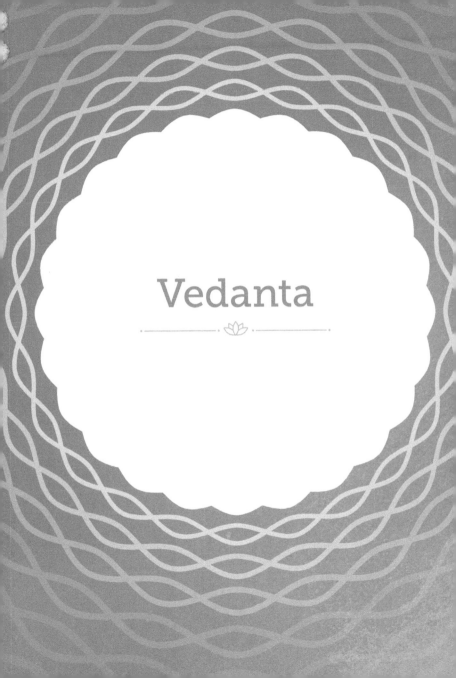

6

Deha
THE BODY

MEANING The body (*deha* in Sanskrit) is one of the three "bodies" (physical, subtle, and nature) to help us function in this world. We have more bodies than meets the eye. *Curious?*

SIGNIFICANCE Our body is our vehicle through which we experience and serve in this life. Thus the reason to make it as healthy, strong, and flexible as possible.

EFFECT You have a body so you can act. Your actions depend on the quality of your mind and intellect: Act selfishly, you suffer; act selflessly, you're free. *The choice is always yours.*

A human being has three "bodies:" the physical body, the subtle body, and the causal body.

1. The **physical body** has the organs of perception and organs of action. The body is what allows you to perceive objects and act in this world. We need to make it healthy with proper diet and exercise. Our physical bodies should be flexible, strong, energetic, active, relaxed, and resilient to disease. These characteristics describe your physical personality.

2. The second body, the **subtle body,** consists of the mind (see page 23) and the intellect (see page 26). It allows you to feel, think, and contemplate what lies within and beyond this world. These capabilities are part of your emotional, intellectual, and spiritual personalities, respectively.

3. The **causal body** consists of your *vasanas*—your inherent nature and innate desires.

Combined, these three bodies are enlivened by Brahman (see page 29) and make the overall personality of you, today.

Surya Namaskar A: Mini Sun Salutation A

Sun Salutations are a great way to start your day! We will do a mini version together.

Come to Samastithi, Mountain Pose (see page 97), a standing position with your arms by your sides. Inhale; extend your arms up and over your head. Exhale; hinge your hips, bending forward, and bring your hands toward the floor. If they don't reach the floor, bend your knees or grab your legs. Inhale; look up and create a flat back. Exhale; forward bend again, reaching the crown of your head toward the floor. Inhale; reverse swan dive, lifting your chest and arms up over your head. Exhale; bringing your arms by your sides for Samastithi, Mountain Pose. Repeat this 3 more times.

> The human body is the best picture
> of the human soul.
>
> —Ludwig Wittgenstein
> PHILOSOPHER

7

Manas
THE MIND

MEANING The ancient Yoga texts describe the mind (*manas*, in Sanskrit) as the house of all our emotions, desires, and preferences.

SIGNIFICANCE The more desires you have, the stronger your mind—meaning the further away you are from your true Self (see page 29). *This creates a more challenging and agitated life.*

EFFECT Depending on the strength of your mind—whether weak or strong—you will either be more free or suffer more, respectively. *Let's weaken our minds to be free!*

The statement about weakening our minds to be free may be confusing because we have generally been taught to strengthen our minds. The difference lies in the definition of "mind."

As mentioned, the ancient teachings define the mind as your emotions, desires, likes, dislikes, preferences, and ego. A strong mind, in this context, means you have a lot of emotions, desires, and preferences controlling you and your actions. What happens when our emotions and impulses take control over us? We suffer and lose control.

How can we not react to our impulsive desires in order to lead a more stable and peaceful life? The teachings explain we need to reduce the power of the mind and strengthen the intellect (see page 26). The mind is neither good nor bad. We just need to understand its nature to gain better perspective of how we got where we are today and how to move forward with wisdom.

PRACTICE

Stand on your yoga mat with your feet together. Set your timer for 60 seconds. Bend your knees and come into Utkatasana, Chair Pose. Reach your arms over your head while shifting your weight back onto your heels. Press your knees into each other. Immediately start to notice how quickly your desires pop into your mind. What preferences arise? Are you wondering when you can get out of this pose? Are you thinking about deepening the pose? What other thoughts arise? Notice the fluctuations of your mind. When you're finished, jot down some notes of your reflections.

The mind is its own place, and in itself
can make a heaven of hell, a hell of heaven.

—John Milton
ENGLISH POET AND WRITER

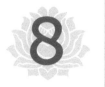

8

Buddhi
THE INTELLECT

MEANING The third equipment humans have is the intellect, or *buddhi*. It is the ability to think objectively and rationally.

SIGNIFICANCE According to Vedanta, the intellect is the only equipment that allows you to decipher between relative and absolute truth—hence, realizing your true Self (see page 29). *Our number one job is to build the intellect!*

EFFECT The intellect keeps us calm and grounded to see the truth and reach our ultimate goal of Self-realization. Strong intellect = peace and clarity.

The main challenge we face with the intellect is that most people don't know they have an intellect, and that it's separate from the mind (see page 23). We think all our thoughts are part of our mind, so it gets confusing and cluttered in our heads.

As you read this sentence, can you hear the words in your head? Most likely it sounds like your own voice. If you're reading this and have an emotional reaction, you're activating your mind. If you're reading this with curiosity and not assigning preferences, you're activating your intellect. Your intellect is your faculty that controls your impulses and desires, allowing you to elevate yourself spiritually and understand what is real and unreal. This generates wisdom instead of knowledge, which is the difference between transformation and information, respectively. *Who's ready to accept that they need help building their intellect? I am!*

Arise, awake, and stop not till
the goal is reached.

—Swami Vivekananda

Set a timer for 10 minutes. Grab your journal and pen. Sit comfortably and close your eyes. Start writing every thought you have without any editing. Do not look at your paper while you're writing. Write without stopping.

At the end of your session, open your eyes and read what you wrote. Can you see the sentences that are emotional and those that are objective? Separate them and notice their different effects within you when you read them aloud to yourself.

Question each statement you wrote to discover what is *relative truth* (that which changes based on personal preferences, mood, etc.) versus *absolute truth* (that which never changes and is constant). You may notice most are relative. *It takes time to look within. Be patient.*

9

Brahman
THE SELF

MEANING *Brahman* is Pure Consciousness. It is the constant, absolute reality enlivening the relative, ever-changing world. *Patience is your friend on this journey.*

SIGNIFICANCE Although it is impossible to understand Brahman with our limited "bodies," conceptualizing can help you see the bigger picture of your ultimate purpose and the true meaning of Yoga. *It's quite humbling.*

EFFECT If you could operate your life from the Self, you'd be peaceful and successful. Eventually, you'd become enlightened and wouldn't need this book. *Then you could teach me.*

Realizing Brahman is the highest—and only—goal of practicing Yoga according to the ancient teachings. Brahman is the same as saying the Spirit, Atman, God, anything associated with the Self, Pure Consciousness, absolute reality, etc. Brahman is what enlivens our body, mind, and intellect.

Compare it with electricity giving energy to a lightbulb, or to the fuel allowing a vehicle to be driven. Neither the fuel nor the electricity is good or bad; it only enlivens the matter to light up or move. Brahman is the same. It is neither good nor bad—it just enlivens everything in the world to live. This is who we really are—our true essence. Yet we are so far away from it because we focus on the body, mind, and intellect instead. It's hard to fathom this could be true. Just the fact that we have stress indicates our separation from Brahman. *Reality check.*

Recognise the unity in diversity.
The one Self pulsating in every facet of life.

—Swami A. Parthasarathy

Experiencing or feeling Brahman is equivalent to becoming enlightened, which neither you nor I are, so there is no way to feel it. There is a mantra, however, that can start the process of understanding the higher knowledge. Mantras are spiritual phrases meant to be repeated in a disciplined manner to help you connect to a higher wisdom. It's important, though, that you don't just say them mechanically.

Choose a daily habitual action, like taking a shower or cooking a meal. While performing the action, see what happens within when you repeat: "I am not the body. I am the Self. I am not the mind. I am the Self. I am not the intellect. I am the Self." At first, it may be easier to repeat it verbally—to hear your voice saying it. Eventually you can repeat it in your head—even while saying something else, you can mentally repeat it.

Identifying with the body, mind, and intellect makes you suffer and become attached. Identifying with the Self—a.k.a. Brahman—is where true happiness lies. As you gain wisdom, you will repeat this naturally.

Bhagavad Gita

10 Karma Yoga
PATH OF ACTION

MEANING *Karma Yoga* is the path of action and selfless service. It's the path to serve with no selfish motive. *Easier said than done.*

SIGNIFICANCE Karma Yoga is the path that helps you purify your body to get closer to realizing your true Self.

EFFECT Practicing Karma Yoga creates feelings of wholeness, compassion, and connectedness to everyone. *Helping others feels good!*

Karma Yoga is the path of action and helps heal the body through higher-quality actions. Everyone must act in this world, so ideally we should act unselfishly and serve beyond benefiting only oneself and one's family. Karma Yoga's purpose is to use the vehicle one was given to serve (the body) to give back to the world without asking for anything in return. One is acting without attachment, giving to be of service and indebtedness to the world, which has given us so much. You gain the attitude of "after you" instead of the selfish approach of "after me." "What can I give?" instead of "What can I get?" People who are both emotional and intellectual in personality benefit from following this path. It's a practical path with a measurable expression. Because we have to take actions every day, we can practice Karma Yoga every day!

No one has ever become poor by giving.

—Anne Frank

Navasana: Boat Pose

Bring yourself into a seated position on your mat.
Lift your legs in front of you and hold your arms out in
front of you for Navasana, Boat Pose. Lift the sternum
and make sure you're at the front of your sit bones.
Keep your knees together and hold this pose for 5 deep
breaths. While in the pose, offer it up to someone else—
for their benefit, their body, their health.

A simple way to feel Karma Yoga is, in traffic, to
let cars go in front of you instead of hurrying to cut
them off. *After you!*

11 Bhakti Yoga
PATH OF DEVOTION

MEANING *Bhakti Yoga* is the path of devotion and love.

SIGNIFICANCE Bhakti Yoga is the path that purifies the mind to help you get closer to Self-realization.

EFFECT Practicing Bhakti Yoga provides you with a sense of humility and a full heart.

Bhakti Yoga is the path that purifies the mind
(see page 23). It's the path of devotion and uncondi-
tional love. When you practice Bhakti Yoga, you
recognize divinity everywhere and in everyone. One
begins to experience a genuine identification with every
living being. No preferential love is felt—only universal
love. Someone who is more emotional will benefit from
following this path because Bhakti Yoga purifies the
mind (the house of our emotions). A sense of fullness,
humility, and deep gratitude is experienced as one
progresses on this path. You have the opportunity to see
the beauty in everything and everyone you encounter
no matter how different. When you see Indians wearing a dot (called a bindi) on the spot between their
eyebrows, that is a symbol of seeing the divinity in the
other that they have themselves. Isn't this a powerful
concept?

Every man is a divinity in disguise,
a god playing the fool.

—Ralph Waldo Emerson

Come to a seated position on your mat and bring the soles of your feet together to touch, your knees bent. Grab your ankles and inhale, lengthening the spine. Exhale; forward bend over your legs for Baddha Konasana, Butterfly Pose.

While doing the physical pose, have the intention of practicing Bhakti Yoga. Connect to the devotion within you by seeing the divinity in yourself and around you. As you bow your head, imagine yourself offering up your practice to something higher and to that divinity. Find some humility in your heart while holding the pose for 10 breaths.

12 Jnana Yoga
PATH OF KNOWLEDGE

MEANING *Jnana Yoga* is the path of knowledge, which requires one to question and reflect on the teachings given.

SIGNIFICANCE Jnana Yoga is the path that purifies and strengthens the intellect through the process of unlearning.

EFFECT Practicing Jnana Yoga helps you witness the world around you and your relationship with it without becoming caught up in it. *Wouldn't that be a blessing?*

Jnana Yoga is the path of knowledge. It's the ability to distinguish between the real and the unreal; the permanent from the impermanent. Consider for a moment what would happen if, in a challenging circumstance, you could be clear on what the truth is and what the truth isn't. You would remain calm because you understood the bigger picture. This is what happens to a Jnana yogi when placed in most challenges. This path requires that you never take anything for granted and that you question everything you've been taught. It's the process of unlearning and relearning.

Reflection is quintessential in this path because it requires your ability to think for yourself. And you can't think for yourself unless you've reflected upon what you've been told to think. It's the path an intellectual personality would benefit from most. This is the path that resonates with me the most because it uses my creative muscle of thinking outside of the box. It's so fun out here!

PRACTICE

Virabhadrasana 2: Warrior 2 Pose

Come to standing on your mat, and face toward the long side of the mat. Extend your arms out parallel to the floor. Separate your feet until they are under your wrists. Turn your front foot to face forward (toward the short side of the mat) and your back foot inward until it is about 60 degrees from your front foot. Bend your front knee until it is above your ankle and keep your back leg straight. Keep your arms extended and engaged. Hold for 5 deep breaths. Inhale; step the back foot forward to meet the front. Switch sides and repeat.

While in this pose, practice Jnana Yoga in the most simplified form. Ask questions to assess what is the best positioning. For example, "Does this feel right?" "Could I adjust something to make this feel better?" "What happens if I do this?"—and shift your feet some. Explore and observe.

13 | Hatha Yoga
PHYSICAL DISCIPLINE

MEANING *Hatha Yoga* is the physical practice of yoga, including the poses, breathwork, and anything that helps create discipline in the body. Think Warrior 2 Pose (see page 42).

SIGNIFICANCE The physical practice of Hatha Yoga can entice the student to learn the other aspects of yoga, including the philosophy. *Consider it the gateway yoga.*

EFFECT Practicing Hatha Yoga makes you stronger and more flexible. It helps you gain confidence while helping you learn to relax.

Hatha Yoga is the physical form of the practice, involving a variety of options relating to healing and purifying the body. You could do yoga poses (see page 95), breathwork (see page 98), and any form of physical discipline. The intention behind Hatha Yoga is to help the student wake up from mundane, routine life to prepare for practicing the three paths of yoga: Karma, Bhakti, and Jnana.

Hatha Yoga alone cannot take you all the way to Enlightenment. It can only awaken and prepare you for the deeper paths of Yoga. Keep this intention in mind every time you go to yoga class or practice at home. You'll ignite the spark within for understanding there's more to Yoga than meets the eye!

Yoga is an internal practice.
The rest is just a circus.

—K. Pattabhi Jois
INDIAN YOGA TEACHER AND FOUNDER
OF ASHTANGA YOGA

Ardha Navasana to Shalabhasana Variation:
Half Boat Pose to Modified Locust Pose

Here's a short sequence to practice daily to strengthen your core (abs and back muscles combined).

Begin by lying on your yoga mat on your back, arms by your sides. Lift your legs an inch off the floor and engage your legs. Inhale; lift your head a few inches, keeping your back on the floor, and look at your toes for Ardha Navasana, Half Boat Pose. Tuck your tailbone under and make your lower back flush to the floor. Hold for 5 deep breaths. Exhale; release.

Flip onto your belly. Interlace your fingers behind your back with your arms straight. Inhale; lift your chest, legs, and arms for Shalabhasana Variation, Modified Locust Pose. Hold for 5 deep breaths. Exhale; release.

Repeat this sequence 3 times.

14 | Svadharma
OWN NATURE

MEANING *Svadharma* means to live according to one's own nature, living your truth. *You'll become a master!*

SIGNIFICANCE When you live your Svadharma, you live in harmony, peace, and acceptance of your purpose regardless of what anyone else thinks.

EFFECT People who decide to follow their true natures lead successful and rich lives. They feel fulfilled every step of the way.

Svadharma translates as one's "own nature."
Sva means "own" and *dharma* means "nature." When one leads a life according to one's svadharma, one lives happily and without resistance. Everything flows.
To know if you're living according to your own nature, assess the decisions you've made. If they're based on your essential nature regardless of what society expects, you're living your full life.

For example, a businessman has thoughts of business and must have a business. Just because you have a business doesn't mean you are natural at business. A musician has thoughts of music and must play an instrument. A teacher must teach. A person who loves numbers and math could go into accounting, engineering, etc. An active, outdoor person must be physical and be in nature. People who follow their nature must be strong and resilient enough to go against the herd instinct. Whoever understands his or her essential nature will be able to serve themselves and others in the most efficient way. This is the only way to live genuinely!

Grab your journal and pen. Answer the following questions as best you can to determine what your nature consists of. You may not have answers to all the questions, but think about them.

- What did you want to be when you grew up?

- What are your natural passions?

- What would you do for work if you never had to worry about being paid?

- What are your first thoughts in the morning?

- What are you naturally good at?

Your primary obligation in the selection of your project would therefore be to find a field you are naturally inclined to.

—Swami A. Parthasarathy

---

15 Paradharma
ALIEN NATURE

MEANING *Paradharma* is living according to one's alien nature. It is a state that keeps us from recognizing our truths and ultimately, Self-realization. This means sacrificing your truth for the sake of laziness, pleasing society, and conforming to the norm.

SIGNIFICANCE When you start your journey toward your spiritual path, you'll hit roadblock after roadblock if you choose according to others' opinions. *You'll feel constant resistance.*

EFFECT While living in Paradharma you will suffer, feel stress, and create pain and disharmony within yourself. You'll find conflict everywhere because you are living in conflict. All your actions will be disingenuous. *You can't live fully this way!*

Paradharma breaks into two words: *para* meaning "alien" and *dharma* meaning "nature"—this means you live or choose against your natural inclinations. For example, if you always wanted to be a singer but went into medicine because your parents wanted that, you would be living your Paradharma. This leads to emptiness, anger, and stress. Everything feels harder to accomplish—you have no energy to complete basic tasks. You live in resistance, because it's someone else's dream or preference—not yours. We choose to live this way because of external pressures from family and society, and because we fear the unknown. This paralyzes us—and it is no way to live. When we recognize this and see the harm it causes, we can take steps toward living in agreement *with* our nature instead of against it. Then you'll live with purpose and be happier. *Let's break out of our Paradharma rut and step into our Svadharma* (see page 46).

If everyone is thinking alike,
then somebody isn't thinking.

—George S. Patton Jr.

PRACTICE

Grab your journal and pen. Answer the following questions as best you can to determine what you've done against your nature or what is alien to your nature. You may not have answers to all the questions, but think about them.

- What did you *never* want to be when you grew up?

- What decisions have you "made" but felt were actually made for you by others, such as your parents, society, etc.?

- Is your current profession one that exhausts you and doesn't fulfill you? If so, why did you choose it?

- What do you dread doing every day because it feels unnatural to you?

16 | **Tamas**
INERTIA

MEANING *Tamas* is the lowest of the three *gunas* (mental states). The qualities relating to tamas are inertia, laziness, and dullness.

SIGNIFICANCE Yoga requires action and Self-reflection—an impossible task while one's mind is tamasik.

EFFECT Tamasik qualities create the effect of lethargy and lack of motivation to accomplish anything. *It's as if your spirit animal is a sloth.*

Every living being consists of the three gunas, also known as mental temperaments. They are tamas, rajas (see page 55), and sattva (see page 58). However, the quantity of each is different depending on the nature of the individual. For example, someone could be 40 percent tamas, 50 percent rajas, and 10 percent sattva. Since tamas is the lowest mental state, it is often compared with the qualities of a rock—inertia and dullness. It's a sense of lethargy and sleepiness with an inability to care about anything.

Although it seems tamas would be a physical quality, it's actually the mind that creates the state of laziness so the body doesn't act. Ideally, where one has tamasik qualities, one would shift them into rajas—activity. Then the ultimate goal is to transition from rajas to sattva—purity and serenity. You will benefit from understanding when and where you are tamasik in your life. *Beat it, tamas!*

My advice is to never do tomorrow what you can do today. Procrastination is the thief of time.

—Charles Dickens
DAVID COPPERFIELD

The "exercise" I'm about to give you is one you've probably already mastered. Sit on your couch. Put your feet up. Grab your remote control, and mindlessly binge watch television. Notice how you feel physically, mentally, and emotionally after spending so much time lazing.

Now try this: Grab your journal and pen, and ignite a bit of rajas to help you out of tamas. Make a list of three areas in your life in which you tend to procrastinate and feel a lack of motivation. Reflect on how you feel daily when you take no action. Then reflect on how you might feel if you decide to stop procrastinating and accomplish your tasks.

17 | Rajas
ACTIVITY

MEANING *Rajas*, the second guna (state of mind), is described as having activity, but with added agitation. *We are making progress.*

SIGNIFICANCE Rajas in motion means we have ignited the fire within to take action, but we remain limited because of our impulsiveness and anxiety attached to the activity.

EFFECT Rajas pulls us out of tamas (see page 52), which is necessary for spiritual growth, but it is also paired with a sense of stress and worry.

We all have a specific proportion of the three mental states (gunas) within us. We can work toward shifting them, depending on the thoughts and desires we fuel. While tamas doesn't care and is inactive, rajas cares too much and is overly active.

Rajasik qualities emerge when we only think about ourselves or our family. This selfishness breeds stress and anxiety. It creates a frenzied form of activity and makes you constantly hurry and run through the day. Visualize New York City streets living in your head. It's frantic and never stops. This temperament makes you exhausted and frazzled.

Ideally, we can elevate our rajasik mental state into a sattvik one by reflection and application of the teachings. Otherwise, one lives constantly agitated and unfulfilled, increasing the level of rajas in our minds. Instead, we should reduce rajas, thus increasing clarity and tranquility. *Chill, rajas!*

Our anxiety does not empty tomorrow of its sorrows, but only empties today of its strengths.

—Charles Haddon Spurgeon
ENGLISH BAPTIST PREACHER

A *Vinyasa* is popularly described as the sequential movements between Plank Pose, Chaturanga, Upward-Facing Dog Pose, and Downward-Facing Dog Pose. A Vinyasa is meant to be one breath with one movement—a breath-movement system of sorts.

On your mat, come onto your hands and knees with your hands under your shoulders. Lift your knees off the floor for Plank Pose. Press your heels back and engage your legs. Push the floor away from you and round the upper back. Make sure your head is lifted. Bring your knees down if support is needed. Exhale; bend your elbows and lower your body for the Chaturanga Dandasana Pose (bottom of a push-up).

Inhale; straighten your arms and lift your chest for Cobra Pose or Upward-Facing Dog Pose. Exhale; press your hands down and lift your hips for Downward-Facing Dog Pose. Inhale back into Plank Pose and repeat 8 times.

Is your mind agitated—either from physical exhaustion or unfulfilled desires? Or both? Just observe.

18 | Sattva
PURITY

MEANING *Sattva* is the highest of the three mental qualities and personalities (gunas). It's described as purity, serenity, and harmony. *Yes, please!*

SIGNIFICANCE Understanding that your highest mental temperament is tranquil and wise helps you see the goal is attainable—it's within you.

EFFECT By practicing sattvik qualities, you'll feel happier, more balanced, and more grounded.

The sattvik state is the highest quality of the mind (see page 23). It refers to a combination of a poised, productive, serene, objective, and contemplative mind. This state of mind is the one we all want to achieve. It means we have developed our intellect (see page 26) enough so as not to succumb to the impulses of the mind, which can be either actively agitated (rajas) or slothfully dull (tamas).

All living beings have a percentage of each of the three gunas. Ideally, one's mind moves from tamas to rajas, then from rajas to sattva. This shows that the mind is evolving because it is being governed by the intellect. Since we all have these qualities, it behooves us to discover how much of each we have. If someone has 100 percent sattva, she would be said to be "Enlightened."

Always aim at complete harmony of thought and word and deed. Always aim at purifying your thoughts and everything will be well.

—Mahatma Gandhi

We are going to practice being poised, serene, and contemplative while holding the Plank Pose. This requires focus, meaning your intellect governs the fluctuations of your mind. *You've got this!*

On your mat, bring your hands and knees to the floor. Extend your legs behind you and come into Plank Pose. Hands are shoulder-width apart and feet are hip-width apart. Press your heels back and press your palms flat into the floor to round your back some. This could create the sensation of pushing the floor away from you. Drop onto your knees for support, if needed. Take 20 breaths and remember to be poised, serene, and contemplative.

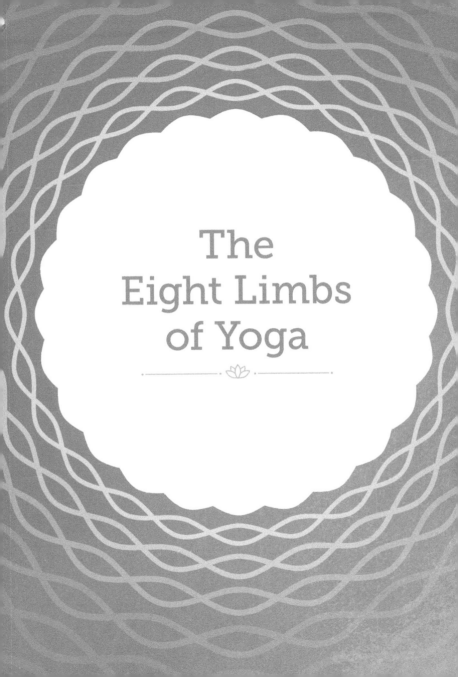

The
Eight Limbs
of Yoga

19

Ahimsa
NONHARMING

MEANING *Ahimsa*, which translates to "non-harming," is the first principle founded in the first limb of the Eight Limbs of Yoga called Raja Yoga. *Confused?*

SIGNIFICANCE If you practice Ahimsa in all areas of your life, you practice Yoga daily; instead of harming others, you are serving others.

EFFECT The physical effects of practicing Ahimsa are powerful—you feel compassionate and connected. This creates a sense of calm and identification with everyone and everything.

Ahimsa is the first principle presented in the five yamas of the Eight-Limbed Path, Raja Yoga. *Yamas* are defined as ethical guidelines. Generally speaking, they are principles that teach us how to relate to others (and ourselves) in a healthy and harmonious way. *Himsa* means "harming" in Sanskrit, and when you place an "a" in front of any word in Sanskrit it translates as "non."

This principle of nonharming teaches us to reflect on where and how we harm others. We can harm with our motives, intentions, thoughts, words, and actions—all of which we have complete control over if we strengthen our intellects (see page 26). We wouldn't even kill a mosquito or cockroach if we practiced Ahimsa fully.

We can also harm by our food choices. I know this can be a touchy subject; try to listen objectively. If we eat animals, we allow them to be slaughtered for the palate preferences of our tongues, which taste food only for a few seconds. We can choose other healthy and balanced food options that don't cause harm to others in the process. *Food for thought.*

On your mat, come to your hands and knees. Place your right knee behind your right wrist for Eka Pada Rajakapotasana, Pigeon Pose. Slide your right ankle toward your left wrist. Slide your left leg back. Inhale; lengthen your spine. Exhale; walk your hands forward and hold for 10 breaths. While in the pose, observe any pain and discomfort that arises. This is a form of harm. Adjust yourself physically so you don't hurt yourself. Observe any judgmental thoughts that could cause you emotional pain. Switch them to positive ones. Observing how we cause harm to ourselves first helps us see how we cause harm to others.

Before you speak, ask yourself:
Is it kind, is it necessary, is it true,
does it improve the silence?

—Shirdi Sai Baba
INDIAN SPIRITUAL MASTER

20 | **Satya**
TRUTHFULNESS

MEANING *Satya*, the second yama, is the principle of being truthful in all areas of your life.

SIGNIFICANCE Without being truthful, one will live a dishonest and delusional life. Continuing in ignorance, we can't get closer to Yoga or our true Self (see page 29).

EFFECT When you practice Satya, you are free because you aren't hiding from anyone or anything. You're living an authentic life to the best of your ability. *Free yourself!*

Satya is the second of the five yamas (ethical principles to follow on how to treat others and ourselves) from the Eight-Limbed Path, Raja Yoga, meaning Royal Yoga. Satya, meaning truthfulness, has many layers. There are lies, deceit, betrayal, white lies, delusion, etc. If we are delusional, we can't be honest. Our perspective is skewed. To gain a greater perspective, we must gain spiritual knowledge. More knowledge eliminates ignorance— the seed of our problems. In the meantime, we need to observe our tendency to tell little lies because we want to be accepted by others and not feel rejected.

From the simple white lie of saying you read a book you never read to something greater, like cheating on your partner, these pull you away from your true nature and create anxiety. Ideally, we would be honest in a way that doesn't cause harm. The truth can hurt but doesn't leave scars, while lies leave marks for lifetimes. *Let's begin to unscar ourselves and others!*

Being honest may not get you a lot of friends but it'll always get you the right ones.

—John Lennon

Utthita Parsvakonasana:
Extended Side Angle Pose

Practicing Satya on the mat means two things: being honest with yourself while in the pose and staying true to the alignment of the pose. Teachers give different alignment techniques. Practice them and see which techniques work well for your body. Challenge yourself wisely. Honor where you are today.

Go into Extended Side Angle Pose: From Sama-stithi, Mountain Pose (see page 97), step the right foot back facing lengthwise to the side of your mat. Extend your arms out to a "T" and separate your feet until your ankles are under your wrists. Swivel your feet to the back of your mat so your right foot points straight back and your left foot turns inward 60 degrees toward the right foot. Bend your right knee so it's above your ankle, and place your right arm in one of the three ways:

1. Place your right elbow on your right knee and left arm over your head.

2. Place your right hand on the floor either inside or outside your right foot.

3. Bind your hands behind your back with your right arm under your right thigh and your left arm behind your back.

4. Take 5 deep breaths and switch sides. Stay true to your alignment and yourself.

When you're honest with yourself, then you can be honest with others.

21 | Asteya
NONSTEALING

MEANING *Asteya*, the third of the yamas, means "nonstealing," and it can be practiced physically, energetically, mentally, and socially. *It's deeper than we might think.*

SIGNIFICANCE If you lived in Yoga (see page 2), you wouldn't feel a void. Stealing implies a void, leading you to seek externals for satisfaction. You'll never find it there.

EFFECT Practicing Asteya makes you the richest person in the world because you always feel you have enough.

As the third principle of the yamas, Asteya serves as a revelation of how we might be thieves—but not in obvious ways. Shoplifting or taking something without permission is the literal form of stealing—but we all steal from nature daily. We take without giving back. Ideally, we would revere what is given to us and not make our lives wasteful. We deliberately serve this world without asking for anything in return. We take, and get upset when nature takes things back through natural disasters. We also take animals selfishly without thought or consideration.

We steal energy from people when we are self-centered and do not pay attention to where we can be of service. Instead, we think about how we can be served. The moment you shift from greed to contentment, you'll never need to steal again. You'll understand the value of nature and animals. You'll feel complete; nature will serve you and provide as needed. Reflect on where else we may steal unconsciously. Me, myself, and mine are our enemies.

Earth provides enough to satisfy every man's needs, but not every man's greed.

—Mahatma Gandhi

Practicing a pose by watching someone else or without thinking it through for yourself is a mild form of stealing. Monkey see, monkey do *not!* You can observe your teacher and learn the general idea of the pose, but you have to come up with your own expression of the pose based on your assessment and understanding. We don't just want to mimic another person without analyzing if that pose works best for us in that way. Find the pose within your body. No two bodies (see page 20) are the same, just as no two minds (see page 23) are the same.

Without looking this up online, read my cues carefully and do your best. On your mat, come to a seated position for Ardha Matsyendrasana, Seated Spinal Twist Pose. Extend your legs straight out in front. Bend your right leg and place your right foot to the outside of your left thigh on the floor—knee pointing up. Place your right hand behind your back on the floor and cross your left elbow to the outside of your right knee. Inhale. Lengthen. Exhale. Twist. Hold for 5 breaths and switch sides. Observe yourself.

22 Brahmacharya
WALKING WITH BRAHMAN

MEANING *Brahmacharya* translates to "walking with Brahman" (see page 29). As the fourth yama, it's the virtue of preserving one's creative (sexual) energy by following the middle path.

SIGNIFICANCE Choosing actions that get you closer to Brahman means you neither indulge in nor repress your desires, helping create an unwavering path to Yoga.

EFFECT Restoring your creative energy brings vitality because it fuels the clarity and peace of mind to stay disciplined on the right path for you.

Brahmacharya, the fourth yama, generally means any actions that bring you closer to Brahman. When presented in the *Yoga Sutras*, it is often misunderstood to mean celibacy, so most yogis abstain from practicing this yama.

Practicing Brahmacharya makes you conscious of how you can overindulge in the sensual pleasures with certain thoughts and actions. These thoughts can lead to feeling forced into abstinence, creating unhealthy repression. Neither extreme uses knowledge to lessen these desires. The mind (see page 23) has complete control, thus depleting our creative, sexual energy. Sex is just one of the main aspects in which we waste our energy by giving into meaningless, habitual exchanges and primitive desires. The idea that "it's not what you do but how you do it" is relevant here because one could abstain from sex but think about it all the time. Is that celibacy? No. We need moderation in our lives to restore, build, and redirect this energy toward something higher, and taper off our lower, sensual desires. *Consider it the ultimate Kama Sutra mental position!*

When you practice Brahmacharya on the mat, you are neither seeking extra pleasure nor suppressing your needs in a pose. Some use yoga to escape reality when it should be used to deal with reality. Find the middle approach, which makes the pose challenging, but not to the point of injury, and relaxing, but not to the point of moaning from pleasure. Practice mentally what you just read while executing the pose.

On your mat, come onto your hands and knees and bring your right foot to the outside of your right hand for Utthan Pristhasana: Lizard Pose. Modify your left leg so it's up or down. Place your forearms on the floor. Your body might jump back and say "too much." You should feel a nice stretch in your legs and hips. Take 5 breaths. Switch sides. Stay centered and don't give in to any extreme desire.

Celibacy goes deeper than the flesh.

—F. Scott Fitzgerald
THIS SIDE OF PARADISE

---

23 | **Aparigraha**
NONHOARDING

MEANING *Aparigraha*, the fifth and final yama, means "nonhoarding." You should not collect nor have possessiveness toward things or people. You can have possessions, but not possessiveness. *There is a difference!*

SIGNIFICANCE Being a hoarder gives you more desires. In Yoga, we reduce desires, especially selfish ones, to live a happier, freer life.

EFFECT When you do not hoard possessions or people, you acquire confidence and contentment. Otherwise, you feel lost and anxious without these things or people.

Practicing Aparigraha, the last yama from the Eight Limbs of Yoga, Raja Yoga, means you understand the lack of security or permanence in the material, including objects and people. When you go shopping, you may feel a need to buy. Most likely there isn't a true need, just a desire. The desire is to not feel a void—so you collect to make yourself whole. It's an illusion of fullness.

Aparigraha is powerful and ironic in that when you no longer have the desire to possess anything or anyone, that thing or person comes to you more. When you suffocate things or people, they want to run away because they feel trapped. Give them freedom, and they come back to you. Reflect on the people in your life who let you be. Do you want to be around those people more or less?

Reflect on the people who call you constantly or demand your attention. Do you want them around more or less?

If our love is only a will to possess,
it is not love.

—Thich Nhat Hanh

PRACTICE

Paschimottanasana:
Seated Forward Bend Pose

Practicing Aparigraha in a yoga pose simply means your desire to achieve a certain pose lessens. The obsession with conquering a pose is replaced with the acceptance that, with practice and dedication, you will get there. Hoarding is a form of addiction, and sometimes one's practice on the mat can become addictive. Let's shift that now.

On your mat, come into a seated position with your legs stretched out in front of you. Inhale; extend the spine. Exhale; forward bend into Paschimottanasana, Seated Forward Bend Pose. Notice your mind's desire to go deeper and reach closer to your feet or beyond. Minimize that desire and get to a 7-out-of-10 intensity. Hold for 10 breaths and release.

24

Saucha
PURITY

MEANING Saucha is the first of five healthy disciplines called *Niyamas* (inner observances). *Saucha* translates to "purity and cleanliness." *Start scrubbing within!*

SIGNIFICANCE Purity is the inner cleanse, while cleanliness is the outer representation of that inward clarity. Toxins thicken your veil of ignorance, making your journey to Yoga harder.

EFFECT Cultivating saucha creates positive energy around you and a hue of beauty, which attracts others to you.

Combining the five Yamas and the five Niyamas gives you the equivalent of the 10 commandments of Raja Yoga in the *Yoga Sutras* (see page 14). VIP note: Yoga philosophy is not a religion. These are ethical, inner observances and healthy disciplines that keep you on your journey to the Self (see page 29). Saucha, being the first Niyama, combines the inner and outer cleanse needed to set ourselves on the path. Your clean and organized house, body, car, etc., represents a clean and organized mind. Your body odor or clothes shouldn't repel others. This is merely the physical sense of cleanliness.

But there's a deeper meaning, too, which involves purity of the mind. The saying, "When the disciple is ready, the guru comes," relates to saucha because a student purified and with a fine-tuned instrument is able to tune into a higher frequency—a guru. *Guru* literally means "remover of darkness," but it is also how we refer to our spiritual teacher. May you be ready soon … if not already.

In the basic sense of saucha, consider how you practice yoga at your studio. Can you make your space cleaner and more pure? Here are some tips:

- Downsize your needs for yoga class.

- Come physically clean and mentally open for class.

- Genuinely acknowledge the front desk person and your teacher.

- Take your shoes off gently and align them in an organized fashion.

- Carefully and quietly unroll your mat while lining it up to the floor and walls.

- Practice each pose with the purest intentions.

Wax on! Wax off!

One must be a sea, to receive a polluted stream without becoming impure.

—Friedrich Nietzsche

---

25 | **Santosha**
CONTENTMENT

MEANING *Santosha*, defined as "contentment," is the second Niyama in the *Yoga Sutras*.

SIGNIFICANCE Yoga and santosha can be synonymous, because when you are content, you do not desire anything more or less. *Ahh*.

EFFECT You feel satisfaction and peace when practicing santosha because you are happy with what you have—and what you don't have.

Santosha is essential for spiritual growth. One's ability to gain contentment is all one needs for happiness in life. Consider the definition of a rich person versus a poor person. It has nothing to do with financial wealth. If your desires are less than the money you make, you're rich. If your desires exceed your income, you're poor. You could have a million dollars, which is enough for your needs, but still feel poor because your desires are greater. Or you could make $100 a week, but if your desires and needs require just $80, you are rich. The person who always feels rich regardless of wealth is content. Joy and gratitude are felt regardless of gain or loss. Practicing santosha means you understand the well-known phrase, "Even this shall pass." You'll embrace what comes and what goes with a smile. *May we all smile at this one day!*

He who is not contented with what he has,
would not be contented with
what he would like to have.

—Socrates

Santosha in a pose can be challenging because we carry negative emotions toward our bodies. We must find acceptance with the body we have. Make the best out of where it is today, and work toward making it healthier for tomorrow.

On your mat, bring your forearms to the floor, parallel to each other for Forearm Plank Pose. Feet are hip-width apart and elbows are under your shoulders. Keep your legs straight. Push the floor away from you and engage your whole body. Hold strong for 20 breaths. You may notice fatigue and shakiness. Do your best and accept your body as it is. The effort is what matters, not the result.

26 | Tapas
SELF-DISCIPLINE

MEANING *Tapas*, the third Niyama (healthy guideline), refers to the ability to practice self-discipline—something most of us lack!

SIGNIFICANCE Tapas requires the use of our intellect (see page 26) to stay on course. *It's easy to fall prey to distractions.*

EFFECT The physical effects of having self-discipline are extreme pleasure in the end, even though it feels like poison in the beginning.

There's a law we all live by, whether we like it or not, which is that whatever is pleasurable in the beginning will be poison in the end, and whatever is poison in the beginning is pleasurable in the end. Consider waking up early to study. Who feels great doing that at the beginning? No one. But eventually it feels great, just like exercise and eating healthy. Consider the opposite. It feels great to party with your friends at the beginning, but in the end, someone gets too drunk or you are hungover the next day. Practicing tapas allows us to stay focused on our path toward Self-realization and Self-development. Cultivate more self-discipline in your life and you will see the benefits, even if is a bit painful to start. *I am your personal cheerleader! Go, Go, Go!*

Self-respect is the root of discipline:
The sense of dignity grows with the ability
to say no to oneself.

—Abraham Joshua Heschel
LEADING TWENTIETH-CENTURY
JEWISH THEOLOGIAN AND PHILOSOPHER

PRACTICE

Here's a self-discipline challenge—both philosophically and physically. Start every day studying Yoga philosophy for 30 minutes, if possible. I recommend *Vedanta Treatise: The Eternities* by Swami A. Parthasarathy, but choose according to your intellect (see page 26).

27

Svadhyaya
SELF-STUDY

MEANING *Svadhyaya*, the fourth Niyama from the Eight-Limbed Path, is described as the ability to self-study and reflect.

SIGNIFICANCE The only way to get to Yoga is to be able to reflect and think for oneself, which is what Svadhyaya requires.

EFFECT By practicing Svadhyaya, you become less impulsive and more introverted, meaning you look for answers within, not from the outside world.

The ability to self-study, Svadhyaya, is vital for the process to Self-realization. You already learned something that you believe to be true. You have to reflect on it and unlearn it to relearn the truth. There are two ways to do this:

1. Question everything you've learned.

2. Never take anything for granted.

By doing these two things, you study how the environment and the information you've been given has formed you into the person you are today. Instead, most of society has been taught to study other people (a.k.a. gossip) and judge. In addition, you have to become a witness (see page 128) to see clearly and objectively. By externalizing our observations, we escape from ourselves. When you can look within, the truth reveals itself.

Did you ever wonder if the person in the puddle is real, and you're just a reflection of him?

—Bill Watterson

CARTOONIST, CREATOR OF *CALVIN AND HOBBES*

With your journal and pen in hand, consider the
question "Who am I?" Write down the first things that
come to mind. Categorize each answer as either being
part of the physical personality, like male or female;
emotional personality, like caring; or intellectual
personality, like smart, etc. Once you've itemized each,
reflect on something deeper within yourself. The process
of Svadhyaya is about the ability to self-study, not
necessarily the outcome. Take a few moments to assess
yourself objectively, as if someone else were observing
you and taking notes. See what surfaces.

28 Ishvara Pranidhana
SURRENDER TO BRAHMAN

MEANING *Ishvara pranidhana*, the last of the Niyamas, is described as surrendering to Ishvara, another name for Brahman or the Self (see page 29).

SIGNIFICANCE Yoga can be found when you have humility; thus the ability to surrender to the higher from a place of knowledge is vital for your spiritual growth.

EFFECT The effects of being humble and surrendering to the Self are inner peace, sense of service, and contentment. *That's a lot.*

Ishvara pranidhana is the Niyama that puts everything into clearer perspective. You are provided everything you need, such as oxygen, light, and food, and ask for nothing in return. When you see your purpose is to discover this true Self by serving and giving back, your only recourse is to surrender to the Divine. We see divinity in everything (see page 37), which fuels a deep love for everything and everyone.

The surrender isn't from a physical or emotional place but rather from a deep-seated understanding that the world doesn't revolve around you, and the world will continue to revolve without you. You must contribute and be of service without selfish motives. Therefore our focus shifts, from obsessing over desires and preferences to the needs of others. With a greater understanding of this truth (see page 40), we act selflessly (see page 34).

PRACTICE
Shavasana: Corpse Pose

Come into Shavasana, Corpse Pose, by lying on your back on your mat. Separate your legs wider than your mat. Turn your toes out. Lay your arms a foot away from your body. Turn your palms up. Make sure your spine is long. As you inhale, think the word "I." As you exhale, think "surrender." Stay in this position for 10 minutes. Set a timer if needed. With every breath, remove a layer of tension from your mind, your heart, and your body. What you are surrendering is your ego, your attachments to your desires of what you want and how you want it. You are here to serve and give back to the Self.

The greatness of the man's power
is the measure of his surrender.

—William Booth
BRITISH METHODIST PREACHER
AND FOUNDER OF THE SALVATION ARMY

29

Asana
PHYSICAL POSTURE

MEANING *Asana*, the physical practice, translates to "seat of consciousness," but it is generally the word used to say "pose." *Strike an asana!*

SIGNIFICANCE Asanas are for a healthy body, but because the physical body is waking up, becoming alert and healthy through the poses, asanas can awaken the other facets of Yoga within us.

EFFECT Practicing asanas feels so good for your muscles because it both strengthens and stretches them. After a solid practice, you feel refreshed!

Asana is the third limb from the Eight-Limbed Path, called Raja Yoga. The *Yoga Sutras* (see page 14), the source that explains Raja Yoga, describe an asana as a steady and comfortable posture. This indicates that every time we do a yoga pose, we should be steady and comfortable—an unreasonable expectation because of our mental desires and habitual physical patterns.

Nevertheless, achieving the poses in this manner is a good goal. Practicing yoga poses is the safest exercise because it uses only your body weight as resistance. You're also holding poses longer than in dynamic exercises, such as aerobics or sports, so you are less susceptible to hurting yourself. In addition, modifications are offered for all body types and situations. For these reasons, all ages can practice the physical postures of yoga. All for one and one for all!

The success of Yoga does not lie in the ability to perform postures but in how it positively changes the way we live our life and our relationships.

—T. K. V. Desikachar
YOGA PHILOSOPHY TEACHER

Stand at the front of your mat for Samastithi, Mountain Pose (otherwise known as Tadasana or Equal Standing Pose). Your toes and heels are touching, if possible. Lift your toes and press your feet into your mat. Engage your quads and lift your kneecaps. Spiral your thighs inward slightly. Tuck your tailbone under. Engage your core. Draw your ribs down and in toward your spine. Pull your shoulders back and down. Activate your arms and fingers toward the floor. Pull your chin in slightly to lengthen the back of your neck, the crown of your head lifting toward the ceiling. Hold this pose for 25 breaths. Look at one spot. Stay steady and comfortable.

30 Pranayama
BREATHING TECHNIQUES

MEANING *Pranayama*, the fourth limb of Raja Yoga, is the practice of using breathing techniques to control and extend the life energy in the body. *Inhale, exhale!*

SIGNIFICANCE *Prana* means "life force energy." Breath gives us this life. We restore our energy to heal the body, preparing it for deeper paths.

EFFECT Cultivating a pranayama practice helps calm your body and mind enough so you can gather a bit more knowledge of the truth through the intellect.

The word *pranayama* can be broken down in two ways: *prana* and *ayama*, or *prana* and *yama*. *Prana* is energetic life force and breath. *Ayama* is to extend and lengthen. Therefore, *pranayama* is the practice of extending and lengthening the energy in the body. *Yama* means to control or harness, so pranayama could also be explained as the practice of controlling the energy in the body. Prana is also breath, so we must learn to control and extend our breathing patterns. Pranayama exercises can be used as an individual practice or in asana practice.

Breath is the only thing that remains present no matter where our minds are. The intellect must be strong to keep your mind on the breath. The problem is, our desires make our minds fluctuate. Hence the reason higher knowledge is needed, so our desires lessen while increasing our intellects. All practices are meant to lead you to the higher, so breathing exercises are only a step toward Self-realization.

Prana is the driving power of the world,
and can be seen in every manifestation of life.

—Swami Vivekananda

The first exercise to learn when starting yoga is Basic Belly Breathing—an optimal way of breathing that provides the most oxygen. It triggers the parasympathetic nervous system, which helps you relax. It's important to master this exercise because all others derive from this understanding.

Sit comfortably on your mat, spine straight, shoulders back and down, chin slightly tucked in. Place your right hand on your belly and left hand on your chest. Close your eyes. Inhale, expanding the belly like a balloon. Don't move your chest. Exhale, drawing the belly in toward the spine, pushing the air out. Keep your chest and shoulders relaxed. Take 20 breaths. As a beginner, never hold your breath. Let it enter and exit smoothly.

31 Pratyahara
SENSE WITHDRAWAL

MEANING *Pratyahara* is the fifth limb of the Eight-Limbed Path. It requires controlling your senses from going outward. Instead, they are pulled within, through greater understanding.

SIGNIFICANCE You can only reach Yoga (see page 2) if you control your mind's impulses and desires, and the constant stimuli entering your body through the senses. *Master your senses!*

EFFECT Controlling your senses, and thus not reacting to the outside world impulsively, means you're becoming more introverted. This means you're calmer and cooler.

Practicing Pratyahara embodies the understanding of the nature of your five senses and your mind. Their nature is to run to externals constantly to find satisfaction and lasting peace.

The problem is, our satisfaction is only temporary when we indulge in the outside world. Our tongue craves delicious tastes even if it lasts only a few seconds, our nose revels in pleasurable scents, our skin seeks a gentle touch, our eyes desire to see beauty, and our ears lean in for inspiring music. Tastes, scents, touch, beauty, and music are all outside ourselves and are subjective. What is beautiful to one is ugly to another. Gaining knowledge helps turn your senses inward and control them. When the tongue desires another chocolate, your intellect says, "Not this time." And so this is needed for all our senses—to be governed by the objectivity of the intellect.

Where the senses fail us, reason must step in.

—Galileo Galilei

On your mat, come to be seated with a straight spine. Pull your shoulders back. Close your eyes. Become aware of your sense of taste. Don't add judgments or desires. Just observe. Take a few long moments here. Then shift to your sense of hearing. Listen without adding stories or flavors. After several moments, shift to your sense of smell. Don't add preferences of like or dislike. Just observe. Then go to your sense of sight. Your eyes are closed, but you may see colors, lights, darkness. Observe objectively. Finally, go to your sense of touch. Notice the clothes on your skin, your hair, a breeze, hot or cold sensations. Don't adjust to make your body comfortable. Notice without attachments or desire. Enjoy your inner show!

32 | **Dharana**
CONCENTRATION

MEANING *Dharana*, the sixth limb of the Eight-Limbed Path, is described as deep concentration toward the highest ideal— Self-realization.

SIGNIFICANCE To practice Dharana, one must significantly reduce desires by gaining a higher knowledge. This provides concentration because of the intellect's development. *Yoga is around the corner.*

EFFECT In Dharana, the physical can't be in tune until the subtlest parts of yourself (the mind and intellect) are finely tuned. The gross (the physical) cannot control the subtle (energetic). *Think about it.*

Dharana requires a higher degree of understanding to get into deep concentration. Pratyahara, the previous limb, is meant to cut away external distractions and desires. Concentration means your intellect (see page 26) is strong enough to keep your mind (see page 23) fixed on one object or thought. The way to achieve this is to negate everything worldly by saying "not this," or "*neti*" in Sanskrit. The process of negation helps us understand that we have to go beyond the pairs of opposites in this world. It's neither good nor bad, hot nor cold, short nor tall, day nor night, etc. What this provides is a real perspective of the absolute truth. Continually keeping this consciousness and strong intellect active eventually takes you to the next limb: Dhyana.

The degree of freedom from unwanted thoughts and the degree of concentration on a single thought are the measures to gauge spiritual progress.

—Ramana Maharshi

Dharana requires a stronger intellect, so instead of sharing something that isn't attainable yet, here are suggestions to help you along. When you're reacting emotionally, ask yourself:

- Can I stop what I'm doing right now?
- Do I want to get out of this emotion and situation?
- If the answers are "no," come back later when the answers are "yes."

If the answers are "yes," ask yourself the following:

- What emotion or thought has taken over me?
- Is it useful?
- What is the unfulfilled desire I have right now?
- What is my intellect saying I should do?

Once you know these answers, consider what action you can take. Then move on.

33 | Dhyana
MEDITATION

MEANING *Dhyana*, the seventh limb of the Eight Limbs of Yoga, is defined as the true meaning of meditation. It differs from the Western approach to meditation.

SIGNIFICANCE Dhyana is an automatic last step on the ladder before transcending into Samadhi (see page 110), a.k.a. the Self (see page 29), a prerequisite to attaining Yoga.

EFFECT Dhyana isn't something we feel physically. It's losing the identifications with our body, mind, and intellect so we now identify with the Self. *Next stop: eternal bliss!*

When the student has been long enough in Dharana (see page 104) by lessening desires so much that only one remains—the desire to realize your true Self—Dhyana is now possible. Nothing more, nothing less.

With your mind fixated on only realizing your true Self, all ego and identification with your three "bodies" ceases. Since you now identify with the Self, you automatically rise into meditation, Dhyana. It's a permanent state, not a temporary one. You can't just practice meditation for 15 minutes daily. Those are simple techniques to help your mind be calm, focused, and relaxed. They are great, but don't get them confused with the true definition of meditation according to the ancient teachings of Yoga. When you're in true meditation long enough, duality dissolves into nonduality (see page 3), and one enters into Samadhi (see page 110).

Trying to meditate with a head full of desires is like a plane trying to take off with too much cargo. Planes must offload the cargo to take flight. Just as humans must offload their desires to be able to meditate.

—Swami A. Parthasarathy
VEDANTA TREATISE: THE ETERNITIES

PRACTICE

Because Dhyana can't be felt or practiced until our desires become exhausted, let's help ourselves reflect on our desires today.

In your journal, make a table with four columns. In the first column, list all your desires. Label the second column, "I must achieve this desire or I won't be happy," and the third, "I can rise above this desire with knowledge and still be happy." The fourth column is labeled, "I don't know yet."

Reflect on each desire you've listed, and check off the appropriate column that suits each best. Revisit and revise the list monthly.

Write the following sentence: "I know I won't be able to achieve meditation until I extinguish all these desires, so I promise to be patient." Sign your name and date it. Evidence of your dedication!

34 | Samadhi
ABSORPTION

MEANING *Samadhi* is the eighth and final limb of Raja Yoga, where one gets absorbed in the nondualistic and highest state of Consciousness. *Enlightenment, baby!*

SIGNIFICANCE Samadhi happens automatically when one has been fully purified by the wisdom gained; it's synonymous with the true essence of Yoga (see page 2).

EFFECT There are no physical effects to Samadhi because it is beyond the physical body. You transcend the identifications with body, mind, and intellect, entirely. *One day…*

Samadhi, the final stage of the Eight-Limbed Path, is equivalent to Enlightenment, thus requiring the practitioner to have no more desires or delusions of the Self. Your single-pointed focus, Dhyana (see page 107), to reach Enlightenment has paid off. The practice of Dharana (see page 104) led you to Dhyana, which led you to Samadhi.

Samadhi is equivalent to entering the fourth state of consciousness: turiya. There are three main states of Consciousness: deep sleep, dream state, and waking state. The fourth state, turiya, is often not discussed. In deep sleep, we wake realizing we felt nothing. That's the best! Reflect on the feeling you have when you wake from a horrible dream and realize it's all a delusion and it dissolves immediately. There's a sense of relief, right? According to the ancient teachings, when you enter the fourth state, you get that same feeling of relief from waking up from the waking state. You realize the waking state is also a delusion and dissolves. *BOOM! Mind blown!*

When the mind, restrained by the practice of
Yoga, comes to rest and when seeing the Self
alone by the self, it is satisfied in the Self.

—Vyasa

BHAGAVAD GITA, CHAPTER 6, VERSE 20

PRACTICE

Since we can't feel Samadhi physically, emotionally, or
intellectually, because Samadhi goes beyond the limitations of language, we might as well prepare ourselves
for it in the future by gaining knowledge today. Reflect
on and study the following phrase. Don't just read the
words, but understand their deeper meaning. In your
own words, write in your journal what you think this
phrase means:

*When the mind, restrained by the practice of Yoga, comes to
rest and when seeing the Self alone by the self, it is satisfied in
the Self.*

A simplified, modernized version reads, "Yoga is the
journey of the Self, through the self, to the Self."

Reflect and see what surfaces based on what you've
already learned in this book.

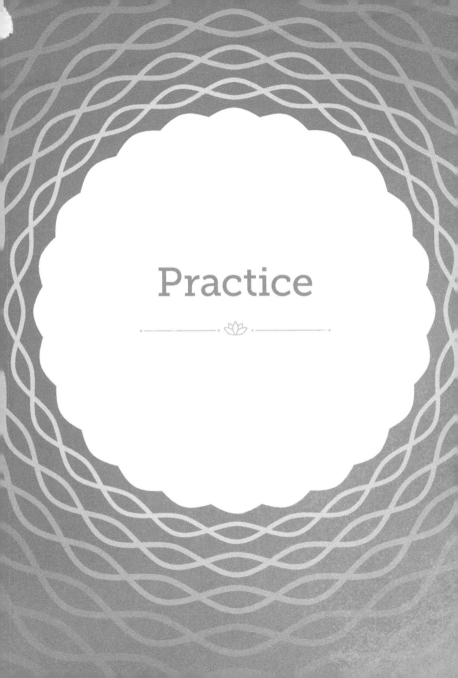

Practice

35 | **Mantras**
REPETITIVE SOUNDS

MEANING A *mantra* is a sound, vibration, or word repeated to focus one's mind (see page 23) on one point so as to connect to something higher.

SIGNIFICANCE Mantras were originally meant to be chanted in Sanskrit, making them more powerful because of their vibrational connections with the Divine.

EFFECT Mantras make the mind calm with the intellect focused on one phrase. As affirmations, they serve to reprogram ourselves. Imagine saying, "I love myself," daily. *What a day!*

Mantras carry a lot of weight because words have power, and we give meaning to those words. Mantras are designed to be pronounced in certain ways where your divine bodily strings are hit to ignite the meaning of the mantra within you. That's their true power.

Another purpose of mantras is as an affirmation, when we need to "brainwash" ourselves away from the negative thoughts we carry daily.

Traditionally, you would chant with a *mala*, a string of 108 beads with a main bead (guru bead with a tassel usually) connecting them together. One hand rests on your knee and the other moves the mala while you chant the mantra—"Om"—and move a bead. "Om" and move the next bead. Continue until you get to the guru bead, then flip the mala around and start over. You can compare it with the physical movement used in moving a rosary, but mantras don't have any religious affiliation. A teacher can show you different ways of moving the mala.

Chanting is a way of getting in touch with yourself.
It's an opening of the heart and letting go of the
mind and thoughts. It deepens the channel of grace,
and it's a way of being present in the moment.

—Krishna Das

PRACTICE

Let's practice chanting a mantra. You can use a mala as described previously, or put a timer on and chant until the timer goes off. Ideally, you'll start chanting the mantra verbally and then make it a silent chant in your head. The inarticulate vibration of the mantra will continue to work. Choose one of the following or choose your own, but don't change your mantra once you begin a session.

- Om Shanti, which means "Peace."

- Om Namah Shivaya, which means "I bow to the divine Self within me."

- I love myself. *You know what that means.*

I have kids say the last one during yoga class, and they love it. As adults, it's harder to say and hear, sadly. Be brave and start loving yourself.

36 | OM

MEANING *Om* is the most powerful primordial sound, or mantra, from which the entire universe becomes manifest, and is the vibratory essence of Brahman, your true nature (see page 29). *Yes, you are that powerful!*

SIGNIFICANCE When we chant Om with devotion, we summon the transformative powers of the word-sound leading to Enlightenment. It is the symbol of Pure Consciousness. *Again, your essence is powerful.*

EFFECT Physically, the effects of chanting Om bring about a sense of peace, harmony, and centeredness. Spiritually, you are attuning with the divine Self within you.

Phonetically, Om is spelled A-U-M. In Sanskrit, the "A" and "U" come together to form the "O." All three together embody the cycle of life and represent the full range of sound. The "Ah" guttural sound represents creation and is formed in the throat where sound begins. *Compare this to the sound you make when you come up with a good idea—"Aha!"*

The "Ooo" (U) sound refers to preservation and travels through the mouth. *When you are figuring out logistics and someone comes up with something enticing, you say* "Ooo." The "Mm" sound represents destruction and is where the lips come together to finish the sound. *When you finish eating something delicious, the final sound is* "Mmm."

Om is an articulate and an inarticulate sound. An articulate sound is one that uses the alphabet and can be understood only by those who speak the same language. An inarticulate sound is one understood by feelings. A laugh in one country is the same as a laugh in another, regardless of language barriers. The physical vibration of Om is articulate and heard by all, while the inarticulate sound is felt once the Om sound stops externally and continues internally.

Om is the most important of all mantras.
All mantras generally begin and often
also end with Om.

—David Frawley
*YOGA AND AYURVEDA: SELF-HEALING
AND SELF-REALIZATION*

PRACTICE
Mantra

Sit comfortably on the floor or in a chair. Place your
hands on your knees. Close your eyes. Take a few deep
breaths. Inhale and say "Aah" for as long as you can
without straining your voice. You should feel the
vibration along your spine and neck. Pause when you're
done. Inhale and chant "Ooo," feeling it in the mouth
region. Pause. Inhale and bring your lips together to say
"Mmm," feeling it vibrate in the crown of your head.
Pause. Take a deep breath in and chant "Ooooom" for
as long as you can without straining. Repeat chanting
Om 10 more times. You may laugh at first because you
feel silly, and that's normal. Rest easy knowing that
chanting doesn't evoke being initiated into a cult.
You're safe.

37

Drishti
GAZE

MEANING *Drishti* translates to "gaze," but it is used externally and internally. It's not only what you see, but how you see it. *I spy with my spiritual eye.*

SIGNIFICANCE The eyes are the windows to our soul, so when we shift our inner vision, our outer vision changes, leading to the truth. *I see you.*

EFFECT Physically, keeping your eyes fixed on one spot helps you stay balanced and centered while in a yoga pose. Cuts away the clutter, if you will!

Drishti is what our sight fixes upon. Literally, keep your eyes on one spot while practicing yoga poses or calming techniques. For example, balancing leg poses can be challenging, but they are easier when your eyes gaze at one point. Gazing is a tool used to help minimize distractions by keeping the mind focused. Your drishti can be placed anywhere, such as up, down, far right, far left, on your navel, your thumb, a finger, your big toe, etc. Each pose tends to have a specific drishti point associated with that pose. When in doubt, your default drishti point is a few feet beyond the tip of your nose diagonally downward. Don't strain your eyes to do this!

Philosophically, your drishti is when your sight is on higher ideals and deeper truths. Change your vision from the external, material world to the inner, transcendental abyss within. This insight is necessary to convert knowledge into wisdom.

No one regards what is before his feet;
we all gaze at the stars.

—Quintus Ennius
239–169 BCE, WRITER

Come into Virabhadrasana 2, Warrior 2 Pose, on your right side (see page 42). Separate your legs wide enough so your right knee is above your ankle when your thigh is parallel to the floor. Extend your arms into a "T," making them parallel to the floor as well. Look beyond your right middle finger, gazing almost at the space around it. Don't look, but see instead. Use your peripheral vision to see the space around your arm as well without moving your eyes. Become more conscious and aware of your surroundings. Sink your eyes into their sockets (I know, sounds weird), and relax your eyes this way. Take 5 breaths and switch sides.

38 | Mindfulness

MEANING *Mindfulness* is the ability to be aware and pay attention to others, your surroundings, and within yourself in the present moment. *Easier said than done.*

SIGNIFICANCE Mindfulness is the temporary state of being present, which requires some development of the intellect (see page 26) so that eventually, with other elements involved, you'll get closer to Yoga.

EFFECT When one is mindful, one is calmer and more peaceful in that moment. It is a skill to develop, so patience is required.

Mindfulness is a popular layman's term for a state of awareness. It's a temporary state that comes and goes as we move from focusing within to becoming externally distracted. Mindfulness is being conscious and considerate of others and yourself without adding judgment or preference. It's a therapeutic term that, ironically, has been used to help calm the mind instead of making it full, as the word implies. Your mind is already full of junk, thoughts, emotions, and clutter.

We need to declutter the mind and slow it down. Therefore, when one is being "mindful," one is actually being "intellectful," meaning the mind is being controlled by the intellect to see clearly and calmly long enough to be in a present space. Ultimately, mindfulness is the beginning step of practicing being a sakshi (see page 128), which is needed in all Yoga practices.

Do every act of your life as though it were the very last act of your life.

—Marcus Aurelius
ROMAN EMPEROR

Get your favorite dessert and put a piece on a fork. Sit comfortably. Keep your spine straight. Grab the fork. Close your eyes. Observe the taste in your mouth *before* eating the dessert. Get rid of any distracting thoughts by focusing on the taste in your mouth. Do this for 30 seconds. Place the piece of dessert in your mouth, but *do not swallow or chew.* Leave it alone on your tongue. Taste the flavor and its sensation for 30 seconds, and then chew slowly and consciously 15 times. Observe while chewing, and swallow. Do this as many times as you need to. Get the sensation of being present for just one moment. That's all that matters.

39 | Sakshi
WITNESS

MEANING *Sakshi* means being a witness, implying we must find objectivity in all areas of our lives. *Observe yourself reading this.*

SIGNIFICANCE The only way to Yoga is to make everything impersonal by becoming a sakshi. This nonattachment helps you gain higher knowledge. *Keep observing yourself.*

EFFECT The ability to become a witness immediately makes you less reactive and more observant.

One of the most powerful tools you can adopt from Yoga philosophy is this tool of becoming a sakshi—a witness. Our days are spent in reaction to outside influences, which makes us deeply involved in and attached to our surroundings. This is exhausting and stressful. Instead, when you can step away from a "personal" situation and observe it from the outside, there is nothing personal about it. We can then find resolution and act consciously.

Consider when you are in traffic: You hate it and react (overreact?) to everything (that person who just cut you off, maybe?). But when you watch traffic from a building, it doesn't affect you at all. This is being a witness. Ideally, you could be in the traffic but see it as if you were in the building so it doesn't affect you. You remove yourself from the situation emotionally in order to intellectually respond in the best possible way, so peace and harmony are cultivated instead of stress and suffering.

One must always be aware, to notice—
even though the cost of noticing
is to become responsible.

—Thylias Moss
AMERICAN POET AND WRITER

PRACTICE

Ardha Navasana: Half Boat Pose

On your mat, lie on your back, your arms by your sides, and lift your legs an inch off the floor. Lift your head an inch off the floor for Ardha Navasana, Half Boat Pose. Take 5 breaths. You will begin to shake and feel the burn. At first you may hate it and want out. Keep holding it and imagine that your witness-Self floats up and watches you doing Half Boat Pose. Stay with me. Hold for 5 more breaths. Notice whether there's a shift from when you were in the pose struggling versus witnessing yourself in the pose. You may still be struggling physically, but there might be a subtle change emotionally and intellectually. Just observe.

40 | **Mudras**
GESTURES

MEANING *Mudras* are symbolic hand, body, or face gestures meant to guide the seeker into bliss and joy.

SIGNIFICANCE The symbolism behind the mudra is more important than the physical gesture. They are handy tools on your path toward Yoga.

EFFECT Practicing mudras calms you and brings you joy while you maintain your gesture and reflect upon its higher meaning.

Mudras are gestures using your hands, body, or face. They are mostly practiced in pranayama (see page 98) and meditation techniques. A common mudra used in yoga is called the Jnana (Gyan) Mudra.

Spread your fingers.

- Your thumb represents the Self (see page 29).

- The index finger is your ego—the individual self.

- The last three fingers represent your three "bodies"—body, mind, and intellect.

When on this path to Yoga, the Self must always be understood as the substratum of all reality. Therefore, our individual self (ego), must always be beneath the Self. This is why this Jnana Mudra curls the index fingernail (your ego) under the thumb tip (the Self), creating an overlapped circle with the two fingers. The last three fingers stay separate from the others because the body, mind, and intellect are not absolute truth. This illustrates why knowing the symbolism behind the mudra you are practicing is important. There's more to mudras than meets the eye ... or hand.

Guided Meditation

Come to a seated position on your mat. Make your spine long. Set a timer for 5 minutes. Place your hands on your knees in Jnana Mudra (as explained on the previous page) with your palms facing up so the backs of your hands are touching your knees. Reflect on the meaning of this mudra. Press your thumb into your index finger to remind you that the Self is above all else and you are not your body (see page 20), mind (see page 23), or intellect (see page 26). Take deep belly breaths (see page 98).

I flipped him a gesture that he wouldn't need sign language to understand.

—Rick Riordan
AMERICAN AUTHOR

41

Bandhas
LOCKS

MEANING *Bandhas* are energetic body locks created to help the yoga practitioner gain a physical lightness in the body. *Sorry, not meant for beginners.*

SIGNIFICANCE Bandhas are another tool for consciously harnessing, increasing, and directing prana in the body to facilitate further development in the practice.

EFFECT Physically, when bandhas are activated, our energy is collected in the torso to build the strength of our vessel (body) from the inside out.

Philosophically, bandha means "bound," implying entrapment to your worldly impressions (*samsaras*). As yogis we are working toward liberation (*moksha*). Physically, the three primary bandhas are:

1. Mula Bandha, the root lock, is the contraction of the perineum, turning the energy upward instead of down and out.

2. Uddiyana Bandha, the abdominal lock, is a suction of the abdomen pulling the energy inward and upward, like a "J" formation up the spine.

3. Jalandhara Bandha, the chin lock, doesn't allow the energy to dissipate through the top but preserves it in the throat and chest.

When all are simultaneously engaged, they form the Maha Bandha, meaning the Great Lock. Engaging Maha Bandha releases stored prana from its associated energy center, letting it flow freely throughout the body. Bandhas are an excellent resource for the day-to-day advancement of your practice.

PRACTICE

Mula Bandha Checks

Come to a seated position on your mat. Cross your ankles in front of your body with your knees toward the ceiling. Place your hands next to your hips. You might need to place blocks next to your hips for extra support. As you inhale, press your hands into the floor (or blocks), and lift your hips off the floor. They may not lift much, but don't be surprised. It takes time to get there.

Engage your Mula Bandha by contracting and lifting your perineum. It's similar to doing a Kegel exercise.

Do the exercise again and lift your hips while holding Mula Bandha and see if there's a difference. Just notice without expectations. Remember, this is a more advanced exercise.

As the mind, so the man; bondage or liberation are in your own mind. If you feel bound, you are bound. If you feel liberated, you are liberated. Things outside neither bind nor liberate you; only your attitude toward them does that.

—Swami Satchidananda

---

42 Pratipaksha Bhavana

SHIFTING PERSPECTIVES

MEANING *Pratipaksha bhavana* is the ability to see things from a different point of view by understanding a higher absolute truth—flipping the mental switch.

SIGNIFICANCE Reaching the state of Yoga requires this fundamental practice of changing perspectives because the sakshi (see page 128) is able to see the truth and quickly apply it.

EFFECT When you practice Pratipaksha bhavana, you feel happier because you see the silver lining in challenges that arise. *Nothing will get you down, because your mind is fixed on the up!*

Pratipaksha bhavana is an instrumental practice in the development of your intellect (see page 26). Simply put, it's your ability to change a negative thought to a positive one. It's easier said than done, because when your mind (see page 23) takes control, negativity tends to take over and drown out the clear, positive voice. With higher awareness and deeper understanding, you'll see the negative thoughts coming and you'll know how to tackle them immediately.

Imagine someone gives you red sunglasses. The world will now look red, but it's only that way because of the lenses on the glasses. Nothing external has turned red, but your perception has changed so you see it as red. The same thing happens when gaining wisdom. You'll be wearing "wisdom" sunglasses, and you'll see the world from an entirely new point of view, even though nothing in the world itself will have changed.

PRACTICE

Sit comfortably. Keep your spine straight. Grab a pen and your journal, and place them on your lap. Set a timer for 10 minutes. Close your eyes and begin to write anything that pops into your mind. Don't edit what comes up. Don't open your eyes while writing. Once you're done, put down the pen and read what you wrote. Notice whether there is a common theme. Do you hear a negative affirmation repeatedly? If you do, shift your perspective on the situation and exchange the negative thought for a positive one. This is the first step toward Pratipaksha bhavana.

Be careful with your thoughts
for they become your words.
Be careful with your words
for they become your actions.
Be careful with your actions
for they become your character.
Be careful with your character
for it becomes your destiny.

—Chinese proverb

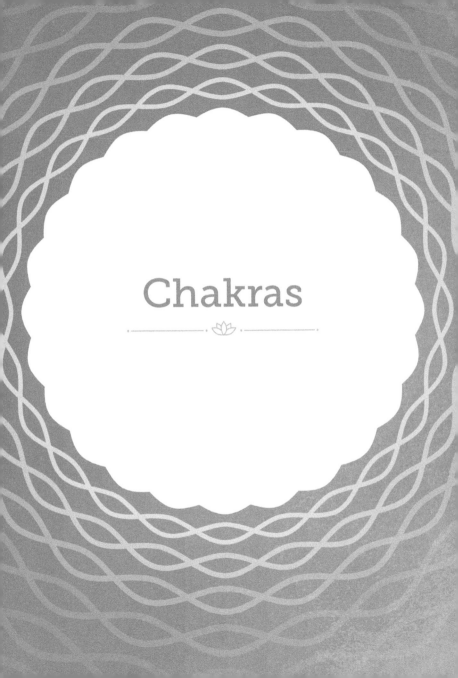

Chakras

43 Muladhara Chakra
ROOT CHAKRA

MEANING *Muladhara*, the first chakra, is also called the root chakra because it's located at the base of the spine. *Are you rooted?*

SIGNIFICANCE Chakras are energy centers in the body—each with its healing function to your spiritual channel within. Muladhara cultivates a grounded and safe relationship with the material world.

EFFECT When you work on healing your root chakra, you feel safe and self-sufficient in the world. *You feel free and stable all at once.*

Chakras are a controversial topic among different philosophies, religions, and studies. Because they are said to be part of the energetic body and physically difficult to prove, there are many interpretations. In Yoga, chakras are part of the Kundalini method, helping you dial into your highest spiritual channel to the Divine by healing each chakra's function and life lesson associated with it.

Chakras are usually referred to as being temporarily balanced or unbalanced in relation to the individual self. Note: People claim they can balance your chakras, but yogis understand we can heal only ourselves. We take responsibility for our lives and empower ourselves. *Who's with me?*

The Muladhara chakra processes our relationship to the physical world, including having our basic needs of shelter, safety, etc. This chakra involves your survival and fear of abandonment by others. Its healing emotion is trust. Think about belief patterns you were taught as a child and that you still live by today. You might be surprised by how much we believe without having thought about it for ourselves first.

Reflect on your relationships with your family. Is there unfinished business lingering? If so, what's stopping you from healing it and moving on?

PRACTICE

Standing poses and balancing leg poses are said to help ignite the Muladhara chakra, but the gross (the physical) can't control the subtle (the energetic). Instead, use these postures to remind you of what relatable lessons still need to be learned.

On your mat, come into Vrikshasana, Tree Pose, by shifting your weight onto your left leg and pressing your right foot onto your inner left thigh, or if you need a modification, put the right heel onto the left ankle and keep your toes on the floor for more balance. Note: Do not put the sole of your foot directly on the knee— either above or below is okay. Make sure you feel rooted. Bring your hands into prayer position in front of your heart. Hold for 5 breaths. Switch sides. Repeat the mantra (see page 116) that resonates best with you: "I trust," or "I am safe."

44 Sadhisthana Chakra
SACRAL CHAKRA

MEANING The *Svadhisthana* is the sacral chakra said to lie between the pubic bone and navel. This life lesson refers to our relationship with sexuality, creativity, and work.

SIGNIFICANCE Because Svadhisthana involves healing our physical relationships, we must heal the one with ourselves first. This creates the life needed to stay on our journey to Yoga.

EFFECT The effects of having a healthy sacral chakra include your ability to create and connect to the power of your sexual energy.

Svadhisthana represents your relationship with sex, money, and creativity. When we haven't learned our lesson associated with this chakra, we create an imbalance. Fear arises of a loss of control or of being controlled by others (for example, addiction, rape, betrayal, impotence, or financial loss). The emotions of jealousy, shame, guilt, and anger reside here when you are in resistance or conflict with others.

On the other hand, if you're healing this chakra, you protect yourself physically and financially. Your relationships are based on your personal empowered truth. You forgive and accept yourself and others. You assert yourself and have control over your body and decision-making power. This manifests into a beautiful relationship within for cultivating creativity and making great things happen. Consider the two things that control most of society … sex and money.

Reflect on how you relate with others. Do you interact in a positive and constructive way, or do you feel compromised?

Remember: The physical poses can't control the energetic body.

On your mat, separate your feet a little wider than hip-width apart and bend your knees so your hips are lower than your knees, going into a low squat. Bring your hands to the floor in front. Repeat the mantra (see page 116) "I create," while doing the following sequence. Exhale; straighten your legs and forward bend. Inhale; bend your knees, lower your hips, and squat. Exhale; straighten your legs and forward bend. Inhale; squat again. Repeat this 8 more times, synchronizing your breath with the movements. Focus on the area between your pubic bone and your navel. *Hint: Follow through on a creative project today.*

45

Manipura Chakra

SOLAR PLEXUS CHAKRA

MEANING The *Manipura chakra* is located in the solar plexus and represents your self-esteem. *We all need more of this.*

SIGNIFICANCE Your ability to believe in yourself helps you stay on course when challenges arise, which we know will be plenty.

EFFECT When your Manipura is healthy, you feel confident and empowered. *Yay!* When it's unhealthy, you feel belittled and rejected. *Boo!*

The Manipura chakra represents the life lessons related to our ego, personality, and self-esteem—all correlated with our personal power.

When unbalanced, we are insecure, lacking self-confidence and self-respect. We live as victims and are unable to take responsibility for our present state. We tend to take things personally and are sensitive to criticism. We live in fear of rejection from all categories, especially appearance issues such as aging and weight changes. Consider where we tend to gain weight— in our tummies, a.k.a. the solar plexus region. Consider whether this could provide insight into emotional imbalances that make us cover up who we truly are.

However, if you are balanced in this chakra, you have confidence, self-respect, and discipline. You'll take calculated risks with effective follow-through. You'll have a strong yet gentle character with a personal code of ethics. When this region is healthy, we know who we are and we don't need anyone to validate us. Think of how much power these principles have over your life.

Reflect on whether you consistently wish your life were somehow different. Have you taken any action to change it? Have you given up and become complacent to your circumstances?

Remember: The energetic can control the physical, not vice versa.

On your mat, come to a seated position and lift your legs, arms by your sides, balancing on your sit bones for Navasana, Boat Pose. Balance here for 5 breaths. Repeat the mantra "Yes I can." On your last breath, lie on your back with your head and legs an inch off the floor for Ardha Navasana, Half Boat Pose. Feel your belly burning. Make sure your lumbar is flush on the floor. Hold for 5 breaths. Now inhale, and lift back up to Navasana. Exhale; lower back to Ardha Navasana. Repeat this sequence 15 times. "Yes I can." Then rest on your back. *It's over. You did it!*

46 Anahata Chakra
HEART CHAKRA

MEANING *Anahata*, the heart chakra, is the fourth chakra and is located in the heart region. It represents the life lesson of cultivating love within.

SIGNIFICANCE Love is defined as a universal identification with all beings instead of a preferential one. When you can experience this kind of love, you have reached Yoga. *BAM!*

EFFECT When your Anahata chakra is functioning, your heart is full and you experience compassion. When it is dysfunctional, you feel hate or grief. *Any takers on the former option?*

The Anahata chakra relates to lessons of love, compassion, and forgiveness.

When it is dysfunctional, we feel resentment, anger, self-centeredness, and an inability to forgive. The fears associated with this chakra are fear of loneliness and commitment and an inability to follow one's heart.

Balance in this region cultivates dedication, inspiration, and the ability to heal oneself. There's an overall sense of nonjudgment and acceptance of yourself and others. *It just feels good!*

This chakra is its most balanced when you are able to be vulnerable with others in a healthy and conscious manner—being yourself and putting yourself out there regardless of consequences or possible rejection. It takes real strength to be vulnerable. This is the simplest chakra to describe, yet the biggest of all the chakras. *Let's heal it!*

Reflect on the people you need to forgive and the reasons you haven't yet done so. Do you somehow like holding onto that pain? Can you let it go?

PRACTICE

Ushtrasana: Camel Pose

Remember: The gross (the physical) can't control the subtle (the energetic).

On your mat, come to a kneeling position with your knees hip-width apart. Place your hands on your hips. Inhale; lengthen the spine and exhale, arching the back for Ushtrasana, Camel Pose. You can keep your hands on your hips, or if you can, place them on your ankles. Lean forward and lift your sternum. Feel the center of your heart opening. Let your head drop back, if possible. Choose the mantra that resonates most, "I love myself," or "I forgive," while taking 5 deep breaths in the pose. Inhale; come back up and bring your hands into prayer position in front of your heart. Repeat this movement 3 more times while opening your heart more and more each time.

47

Vishuddha Chakra

THROAT CHAKRA

MEANING *Vishuddha*, the fifth chakra, is located in the throat region and represents one's will, self-expression, and ability to communicate truthfully. *Find your voice.*

SIGNIFICANCE Developing your will and self-expression is vital to thinking and speaking up for yourself. Following the herd won't get you to Yoga.

EFFECT The effects of speaking freely and openly create a conscious freedom to vocalize your truth without justification. No more silencing, hiding, or running away.

The Vishuddha chakra represents your choice and strength of will, your personal expression, and your ability to communicate clearly and truthfully—both verbally and nonverbally. When the chakra is dysfunctional, it can manifest as shyness, gossip, lying, or an inability to make a decision. The fear of having no authority or power of choice in your life arises in this chakra. There is also a fear of surrendering your power to the divine without fully understanding the concept and reason.

When this chakra is functional and healthy, it provides personal authority, honesty, and keeping your word to others and yourself. We communicate in many ways; if you are thinking and feeling one thing but communicating another, you are not in balance. There is a blockage that needs to be evaluated and healed. Communicating with conviction, clarity, and compassion is the result of working through your blockages.

Reflect on your ability to communicate honestly, openly, and directly. If you find you cannot, consider when it happens and the possible reasons for it.

Remember: This pose can't help you heal the subtler areas within.

On your mat, lie on your back with your legs out straight. Grab your outer thighs and press your elbows into the floor. Lift your chest and arch your head back until the crown of your head hits the floor for Matsyasana, Fish Pose. Mentally repeat the mantra "I am truthful," or "I speak up for myself." Choose the one that resonates with you. Feel your throat open and breathe deeply. Engage your legs and make sure you're still pressing your arms down so you do not collapse your neck. Take 5 deep breaths and reflect on the mantra. Repeat the pose 3 more times.

48 | Ajna Chakra
THIRD EYE CHAKRA

MEANING The *Ajna* chakra, energetically located between the eyebrows, is the sixth chakra. It represents your insight, wisdom, and developed intellect.

SIGNIFICANCE This chakra is essential to transforming your knowledge and random, undigested information to wisdom and calculated, digested truth, thus bringing you closer to Yoga.

EFFECT The Ajna chakra is your spiritual eye chakra (third eye chakra), which helps you see clearly when functioning optimally. When dysfunctional, it keeps you in ignorance. *No thank you.*

The Ajna chakra's function is related to one's intuition, wisdom, and insight.

The lessons to observe are your ability to self-evaluate, to question, and to think for yourself. The insight associated with this chakra helps you listen to others' ideas objectively without adding skewed judgments or personal interpretations. A fear related with this chakra is our fear of looking within. This creates even more fears, because without looking within, your intellect is too weak for the discipline needed to evolve. Then the mind is too strong and we are afraid of our shadows, our darker places within—which we all have.

When functioning smoothly, this chakra brings the most important function a human could develop: the intellect (see page 26). You feel inspiration to act from creativity, intuition, and reasoning—the trio necessary on the journey to your inner treasure!

Reflect on the attitudes and beliefs you would like to change within yourself. Are you willing to do what it takes to make those changes?

On your mat, come onto your hands and knees. Sit back on your heels for Balasana, Child's Pose. Make sure your third eye, the spot between your eyebrows, touches the floor, or a pillow if you need support. Bring your arms by your sides to relax entirely in the pose. If your bodyweight is pushing you forward, keep your arms in front for support. Put all your attention on the spot between your eyebrows and repeat the mantra "I am willing to go within for my answers." Hold for 5 minutes, if it's relaxing, while repeating the mantra and focusing on your third eye. Resist the resistance to look within.

49

Sahasrara Chakra

CROWN CHAKRA

MEANING *Sahasrara*, the seventh chakra, is located on the crown of the head and represents our connection to the Divine. *Hello, Divine. Anyone home?*

SIGNIFICANCE The crown chakra keeps us true to our higher ideals, the purpose behind healing all the chakras and studying the practice of yoga. It comes full circle.

EFFECT When this chakra is balanced, you feel connected and have a higher purpose. When it is unbalanced, you're attached to this world and feel alone.

The Sahasrara chakra is related to our spirituality, meaning our divine wisdom and the integration of the physical self with the higher Self. The overall lessons in this chakra are the ability to trust life, to be selfless (devoid of ego), and to be devoted to Brahman (see page 29). Devotion is often misconstrued when misunderstood. Think Bhakti Yoga (see page 37).

The fears in this chakra are of feeling a loss of identity and a loss of connection with life, beings, and the people around us. Spiritual abandonment is felt when the crown chakra is unbalanced. This can create the susceptibility to fall to the "dark side," giving in to your shadows, so that the mind (see page 23) completely takes over. No wisdom can be gained here.

On a lighter note ... if this chakra is balanced, you have a higher understanding of Brahman, helping you feel connected to all beings—giving you faith in the larger picture of this crazy and beautiful life we live. *A light at the end of the tunnel!*

Reflect on the times you've tried going deeper within yourself but stopped. Why did you stop? Can you start a practice that helps you continue this process?

To feel Sahasrara chakra, you must do a perfect head-stand. Just kidding! Remember, these physical poses can't control the subtler aspects of your existence. They are just symbolic of something deeper, which we connect to by adding mantras or intentions.

Instead of a headstand, we will do my favorite supported inversion: Legs Up Against the Wall Pose. Find a wall where you can lie on your back with your buttocks touching the wall and your legs extended upward. Make sure your sitting bones are flush to the wall and your back is flat. Relax your arms by your sides. Repeat the mantra that suits you: "I am connected," or "I am devoted." Hold for 10 minutes. Relax as much as possible and take deep breaths.

Hatha Yoga Styles

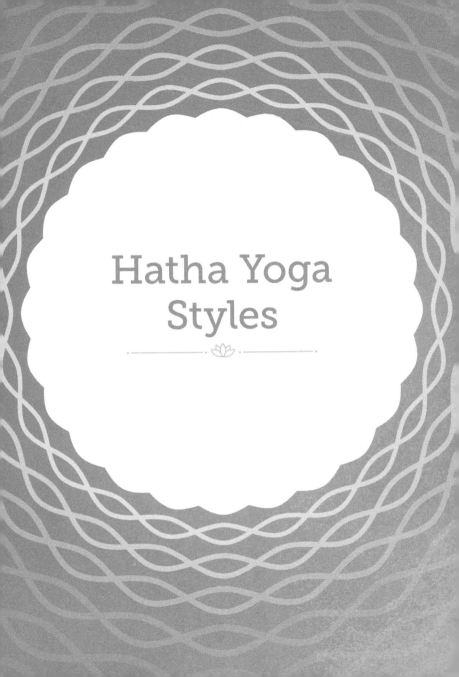

50 Ashtanga Vinyasa Yoga

MEANING *Ashtanga Vinyasa Yoga* is a style of Hatha Yoga (see page 43) that originated in India. It was created by K. Pattabhi Jois in 1948 and is known for its repetitive sequences, adjustments, and intensity. *Great for Type-A personalities!*

SIGNIFICANCE Ashtanga Vinyasa Yoga is one of the yoga styles that became mainstream and popular in the West because of its physically challenging nature.

EFFECT Ashtanga Yoga is physically demanding because of the *Vinyasas*, or dynamic stretching. Vinyasa means "breath with movement," so for each movement there is one breath.

K. Pattabhi Jois, who designed Ashtanga Vinyasa Yoga, was one of Krishnamacharya's disciples, based in Mysore, India. Krishnamacharya was a yoga teacher and scholar responsible for awakening Hatha Yoga in the West and is known as the Father of Modern Yoga.

Ashtanga Yoga consists of six series with different intentions. They are set sequences with a strict rule that a student can't go to the next pose in the sequence unless the teacher approves. Also, the student can't go out of sequence order. Its main focus is on Vinyasas, Ujjayi breath, Bandhas (see page 134), and Drishti (see page 122).

The Primary Series, also called Yoga Therapy, is challenging and meant for a certain kind of flexible hip—one most Westerners don't have because we sit in chairs instead of squat on floors. The style calls for two things, which eventually are the reasons it declined in popularity—alignment that is not traditionally taught and intense and aggressive adjustments.

This combination created a lot of injuries, and students found alternatives. Thus the birth of Vinyasa Yoga, Power Yoga, Rocket Yoga, and similar styles, which gained traction. Teachers morphed Ashtanga's strict and elite sequences to more forgiving and fun ones for Western bodies and lifestyles. Ashtanga was my first practice, and for that I am forever indebted!

Do your practice and all is coming.

—K. Pattabhi Jois

PRACTICE

If Ashtanga Vinyasa Yoga is your choice of physical yoga, as a beginner, I would find a teacher who helps you into the poses safely. You'll learn Sun Salutation A and Sun Salutation B, then some of the standing poses like Triangle Pose, Twisted Triangle Pose, Side Angle Pose, Twisted Side Angle Pose, and Extended Forward Bend Pose. With a qualified teacher who understands each student's boundaries, you can go farther.

Hint: Don't study with a teacher who adjusts you too much. It's best to learn the poses on your own first with only minor adjustments.

Keep these five tips in mind for all standing poses:

1. Push the floor away from you with your feet. Don't let gravity win.

2. Engage your quads by lifting your kneecaps.

3. Engage your core.

4. Lengthen your spine.

5. Learn how to breathe Ujjayi breath.

51 | Iyengar Yoga

MEANING *Iyengar Yoga* is a style of Hatha Yoga (see page 43) created by B. K. S. Iyengar from India. It is known for its attention to alignment. *Great for perfectionists!*

SIGNIFICANCE Iyengar Yoga became mainstream in the West about the same time as Ashtanga Yoga (see page 166) but focused on alignment, holding poses, and using props. *Adaptable for all bodies.*

EFFECT One who practices Iyengar Yoga knows all too well how hard it is to hold not just the body, but also the mind, in one position—a.k.a. static active stretching.

B. K. S. Iyengar was another of Krishnamacharya's disciples, although the style of Hatha Yoga he created is very different from that of K. Pattabhi Jois (see page 166). In fact, it seems like they decided on two opposite methods when it came to the physical practice. My Jnana Yogi wonders how that came about from having the same teacher. Luckily, the answer is simple: There are different practices for different personality types. Depending on your personality, you will gravitate toward one style of yoga over another. Neither one is good or bad, just right or wrong for a particular person.

Iyengar Yoga claims to have a therapeutic approach because of its use of props, alignment, and the long time spent in a pose. The props used during practice include straps, bolsters, blocks, blankets, the wall, chairs, etc. The intention behind this is to prevent injuries due to straining beyond one's physical capacity. These props assist beginners to accomplish the poses safely and eventually not to need the props once the poses are mastered. *Grab your blocks, beginners!*

Paschimottanasana: Seated Forward
Bend Pose, with props

Grab a blanket and a strap or a belt. Fold the blanket
and place it on the floor. Sit on the blanket's edge so
your hips rotate forward. This helps with tight hips.
Extend your legs in front of you for Paschimottanasana,
Seated Forward Bend Pose. Put the strap around the
balls of your feet and gently pull on it help to relieve
tight hamstrings. Inhale; extend the spine and keep it
straight no matter what. Exhale; hinge the hips and
lower your torso without rounding your back. Pull
forward as you exhale into the pose. Engage your quads,
take deep breaths, and hold this pose for a long time—
until it feels like longer than forever!

Yoga teaches us to cure what need not be
endured and endure what cannot be cured.

—B. K. S. Iyengar

52 | Restorative Yoga

MEANING *Restorative Yoga* is a therapeutic form of passive static stretching where props are used to support the body and help it stretch without engaging muscles. *It's so yummy.*

SIGNIFICANCE While Ashtanga Yoga and Iyengar Yoga both require more physical exertion, Restorative Yoga is ideal for relaxing by learning how to surrender and let go. *It's soo yummy.*

EFFECT Restorative Yoga teaches you to relax and destress by finding value in the disengagement of muscles. You feel refreshed and renewed. *It's sooo yummy.*

Restorative Yoga is exactly what the name implies— yoga that restores your energy by tapping into a deep relaxation, which triggers healing. It helps increase flexibility, reduce stress, and boost your immune system. It originated from Viniyoga, a therapeutic style of yoga founded by T.K.V. Desikachar, Krishnamacharya's son and disciple. Your parasympathetic nervous system kicks in, which disables your fight-or-flight response (sympathetic nervous system) generated from daily challenges. While practicing this, you must surrender and have enough control over your muscles to let them disengage.

With the use of props, all body types can find a comfortable position to hold for a long time to deepen the stretch safely. You'll identify, rather quickly, where you hold tension, those areas where you feel resistance. This style of yoga is great for beginners because it helps them connect with their bodies in a gentle, compassionate way. As a student, you want to create a range in your practice by doing both the more intense yoga styles and the more relaxing ones. This way you don't become attached to one form, but continue to evolve as a diverse being. Plus, did I mention that it's soooo yummy?

Grab two bolsters and three blankets. Place one bolster lengthwise on your mat so the long side is parallel to the side of your mat. Place an additional bolster horizontally across the first bolster to create a "T." Sit facing away from the bolsters so the bottom of the "T" is touching your sacrum. Lean back onto the bolsters so your spine is on an incline. Place the soles of your feet together and let your knees fall apart for Viparita Baddha Konasana, Reclined Butterfly Pose.

Place the blankets under your thighs so your knees are lifted slightly. You can put a blanket over you to remain warm, if you wish. Arms are open to the sides for a chest and shoulder stretch. Breathe deeply and hold here for 5 to 10 minutes.

The quieter you become
the more you are able to hear

—Rumi
THIRTEENTH-CENTURY POET

GLOSSARY

ARJUNA: The warrior in the Bhagavad Gita chosen to lead the fight for the righteous Pandava royal family and against the unrighteous Kauravas royal family because they were destroying the kingdom. He collapsed at the beginning of the battle, unable to fight until he asked for Krishna's help.

ATMAN: Ancient yoga texts give many names to the same principle, thus Atman is another word for Brahman, Pure Consciousness, Spirit, God, and the Self.

CHAKRA: Translates to "wheel" or "disk." Chakras are energy centers in the body relating to respective life lessons that need to be learned and healed.

GURU: A spiritual teacher. Literally translates into "remover of darkness."

JALANDHARA: *Jala* means "net" and *dhara* means "stream" or "flow"; one of the three main Bandhas.

KRISHNA: An embodiment of Brahman and Arjuna's guide in the battle for righteousness. Arjuna's collapse leads to an opening for Krishna to reveal to him the real truth about life. He gives the sermon and lets Arjuna decide for himself what is needed.

MAHABHARATA: The epic tale written by sage Vyasa depicting the story of two royal families—the Pandavas and the Kauravas. The Bhagavad Gita is embedded into the *Mahabharata* and teaches the philosophy as part of the tale.

MULA: Translates to "root" or "base"; one of the three main Bandhas.

NIYAMA: The second limb of Raja Yoga, offering healthy disciplines one should acquire as daily practices toward Enlightenment.

RAJA YOGA: The Royal Path of Yoga, also known as the Eight Limbs of Yoga, consisting of guidelines for students to practice to reach the highest level of Consciousness.

SAMASTITHI: *Sama* means "equal" and *stithi* means "standing." Samastithi is a principle to apply in your yoga practice by equally engaging in all the poses. It's also another name for Tadasana, or Mountain Pose.

SWAMI: A highly respected title for an Indian master who specializes in philosophy and yoga.

SWAMIJI: *Swami* is a highly respected title for a spiritual teacher and *ji* means beloved, so when you combine the two words *Swami* and *ji* together, you are saying "beloved teacher." You can combine *ji* with names, too. Saying "Rinaji" would mean "beloved Rina," for example.

UDDIYANA: Translates to "upward lifting" or "flying upward"; one of the three main Bandhas.

UJJAYI: An audible breath used to trigger the parasympathetic nervous system in the body, while also heating up the body from the inside. It sounds like the ocean (or Darth Vader).

VASANAS: One's innate nature or natural inclination; also considered to be one's consistent desires.

VINYASA: *Vi* means "in a special way" and *nyasa* means "to place," so together they mean to "place in a special way"; used popularly to describe the sequential movements between Plank Pose, Chaturanga, Upward-Facing Dog Pose, and Downward-Facing Dog Pose. It is meant to be one breath with one movement—a breath-movement system of sorts.

YAMAS: The first limb of Raja Yoga offering ethical guidelines and principles on how to relate on a higher level to others on a daily basis.

PHILOSOPHY SCHOOLS

CHOOSING THE RIGHT SCHOOL AND TEACHER FOR YOU

Throughout my years seeking a teacher, I easily found books on Yoga philosophy, but it was not as easy to find well-rounded, thorough philosophy schools dedicated solely to this cause. A lot of yoga schools and centers have different programs and teachers from various lineages and lifestyles. Although this may benefit those who like variety, it's not optimal for those of us who need a disciplined, focused, foolproof path.

So instead of sharing teachers and schools here that I've never had personal experiences with (*both for liability purposes and to remain authentic*), I highlight how to find the right teacher and school for yourself.

Choose a teacher or school that:

- Lets you think for yourself and encourages questioning.
- Never imposes their beliefs or opinions on you.
- Preaches what they practice, meaning they are the example behind what you are learning.
- Has a lineage and sources to the teachings you're studying.
- Is accessible and allows you time with the teacher when requested.
- Uses logic and reasoning.
- Knows how to set healthy boundaries in a teacher/student relationship without touching you inappropriately or making you feel uncomfortable.
- Helps you evolve and grow, as proven by your ability to handle life's challenges gracefully.

Learning About Vedanta

School: The Vedanta Academy in India

Teacher: Swami A. Parthasarathy (b. 1927–)

Principal Beliefs: This academy's sole purpose is to help develop the student's intellect, not intelligence. It runs 365 days a year with no weekends or holidays.

Resources:
- Books to read, in this order (all by Swami A. Parthasarathy):
  The Fall of the Human Intellect
  Governing Business and Relationships
  The Holocaust of Attachment
  Vedanta Treatise: The Eternities
- Three-year online course
- Three-year course at the Academy in India
- Website: www.vedantaworld.org
- Vedanta Schools in the United States:
  Vedanta Institute of Los Angeles, www.vedantala.org
  Vedanta Institute of Malibu, www.vedantamalibu.org
  Vedanta Institute of New York, www.vedantausa.org

Learning About the *Yoga Sutras of Patañjali*

School: Satchidananda Ashram in Yogaville (Virginia)

Teacher: Swami Satchidananda (1914–2002)

Principal Beliefs: From the *Yoga Sutras of Patañjali*. Although I have not studied at the ashram as a student, I have had the pleasure of teaching both philosophy and physical yoga there and had a wonderful experience! I have also thoroughly read the *Yoga Sutras of Patañjali*, and it gave me a foundation to tackle Vedanta when it finally crossed paths with me many moons later.

Resources:
- Book: *Yoga Sutras of Patañjali*
- Website: www.yogaville.org or www.swamisatchidananda.org

RESOURCES

BOOKS

Hay, Louise. *You Can Heal Your Life*
Although this book is not directly about Yoga philosophy, it does provide insight into how the subtle body controls the physical body. In order to build one's intellect, we need to address the issues preventing us from moving forward on our spiritual path.

Hoff, Benjamin. *The Tao of Pooh*
This is a good beginner's book for understanding a new perspective on our way of life. It's written as a simple Winnie the Pooh story, yet so clearly explains the direction we should all choose for a peaceful life.

Myss, Caroline. *Anatomy of the Spirit*
If you're interested in learning more about the chakras, this book gives the perspective of balancing your chakras to heal your life. It provides powerful, probing questions for the reader to reflect on.

As noted in the Appendix, page 183, Parthasarathy's books should be read in the order listed:

Parthasarathy, A. *The Fall of the Human Intellect*
This book is a great start to your journey to building your intellect. A. Parthasarathy suggests reading this book first to get your feet wet for the rest of the denser information that comes in the following books.

Parthasarathy, A. *Governing Business and Relationships*
If you work or relate with others (mostly everyone), this book is a great help in understanding why you fail and gives you clear guidance on how to succeed.

Parthasarathy, A. *The Holocaust of Attachment*
Presents a look into the deadliest disease we all carry—attachment. This book is for those with thicker skin willing to hear the truth and reflect upon it more deeply.

Parthasarathy, A. *Vedanta Treatise: The Eternities*
This is the mother of all Yoga philosophy texts and a user-friendly manual to your life. From A to Z, it provides everything you ever wanted to know about the path toward Self-realization. If you only have time to read one of the four books suggested, then read this one!

Parthasarathy, A. (translator). Bhagavad Gita

There are many translations and commentaries of the Bhagavad Gita, but this one provides the most logical conversational tone. It's easy to follow and holds the reader's hand through something that is dense in nature.

Satchidananda, Swami (translator; commentary by). *Yoga Sutras of Patañjali*

This book is written in layman's terms to provide an understandable explanation of *Yoga Sutras of Patañjali.*

MOVIES

I Heart Huckabees

This movie does a wonderful job of showing the intricacies of the teachings, such as delusion and the Self in a visual form. It doesn't implicitly state a reference to Yoga teachings, but they are embedded deeply—pay close attention.

Peaceful Warrior

For us visual learners, this movie displays some of the principles of Yoga, like referencing the ego, the teacher within, being present, etc. You'll have to connect the dots yourself after studying the principles.

Vedantaworld.org

This website provides video lectures and an online philosophy course by A. Parthasarathy and Sunanda Leelaram (A. Parthasarathy's daughter). They are presented in conversational tones and provide visual learning, which can be more effective for some. Hearing and watching the source speak can be a powerful form of transference.

INDEX

ACKNOWLEDGMENTS

Thank you for the many blessings and serendipitous moments that had to connect to make this book happen.

My first blessing is my dear husband, Eric Paskel (EP), for changing the course of my life by introducing me to the one and only Swami A. Parthasarathy, and for filling my days and nights with true love, explosive laughter, and EPisms.

My second blessing is Swamiji himself, for taking the time to study and share these sacred teachings with spiritually hungry students like me.

The third blessing is my team at Callisto Media, Inc. Brian Hurley, for the long and trustworthy leash you gave me to write this book and for our clear and collaborative communication. And to my efficient and calm editor, Mary Cassells, for helping my words come to life in a whole new way and for your meticulous attention to detail.

Last, but not least, is my fourth and forever blessing of my parents, for always believing in me and supporting me in everything I do. I'm forever indebted to you all and am humbly bowing to you as I write these words. Namaste.

ABOUT THE AUTHOR

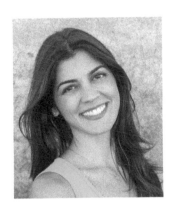

Rina is full of life, love, and imagination!

Rina Jakubowicz is known for her vibrant and uplifting approach to yoga and life. She is an international bilingual yoga teacher, Reiki practitioner, motivational speaker, and author. She has been a teacher of teachers since 2005, presenting at *Yoga Journal* conferences, Himalayan Institute, Omega Institute, Kripalu Center, and Wanderlust Festivals, as well as in countries across the globe such as Chile, Puerto Rico, Mexico, and Andorra.

You can practice with Rina online on Gaia TV, Shri TV, and Yogis Anonymous. She's the yoga expert on Univision's Tu Desayuno Alegre and a regular contributor to Yoga Journal Online and MindBody-Green. She's appeared on the cover of *Yoga Journal* several times in the United States, been featured in their Spain and Russia issues, and graced the cover of Canada's *Sweat Equity*.

You can see Rina in *NY Yoga+Life Magazine*, *Origin* magazine, *Mantra* magazine, *Glam Belleza Latina*, and *Revista Mujer*, among other publications worldwide.

Rina currently lives in Los Angeles, California, although her hometown is Miami, Florida. She founded Rina Yoga studios in Miami in 2005 and was selected as one of South Florida's Business Leaders Movers and Shakers in 2011. She also created the yoga app Snooze Yoga and a pioneering yoga curriculum for children and teens called Super Yogis' Schoolhouse.

Printed in the USA
CPSIA information can be obtained
at www.ICGtesting.com
CBHW040307050324
4972CB00013B/99